MARIO BADESCU'S
SKIN CARE PROGRAM FOR MEN

Mario Badescu's Skin Care Program for Men

BY MARIO BADESCU

Illustrations by John Gampert

EVEREST HOUSE *Publishers, New York*

Library of Congress Cataloging in Publication Data:
Badescu, Mario.
    Mario Badescu's skin care program for men.
    1. Skin—Care and hygiene. 2. Grooming for men.
I. Title.
RL87.B29   1980   646.7'26   80-13213
ISBN 0-89696-032-3

To America, my adopted homeland,
in gratitude for the freedom, good fortune,
and happiness I have found here

CONTENTS

PREFACE

I HAVE been a skin-care specialist for the last twenty-five years, first in my native Romania, then in Vienna and, since 1965, in New York. Throughout my career, I have watched trends—psychological as well as chemical—in skin care closely. And frankly, even I could not have predicted, say, ten years ago, that men would be paying as much attention to their skin as they are doing today. As recently as the early Seventies, skin was still a topic at home only in the health and beauty pages of the women's magazines.

Women—at least the *smart* women—have long been aware that how their skin looked not only influenced how they appeared to others on a superficial, first impression level, but that it could confer real psychological benefits as well. Skin that was clear, translucent, free from blemishes enhanced their self-esteem, made them *feel* good. Just as important, many of them understood that skin condition was a direct reflection of actual body health, of metabolism and energy level, of various systemic dysfunctions, of anxiety or the absence of anxiety.

But until very recently almost no man realized any of this, mostly because no man was made aware of the benefits of good skin care. Shaving in the morning and lamenting the occasional pimple were as much as he had been educated to do. Then several things happened, virtually all at once. First, the entire country became fitness-minded. Health-club memberships, running and jogging shoe sales, and mineral water consumption doubled, then doubled again. We were catapulted into what one writer later dubbed the "Me" decade, and a healthy body was central to active, successful participation in it.

Simultaneously, men were encouraged to think seriously about how they looked, in part as a result of their new concern for their bodies, in part as a result of new standards of masculinity—more relaxed, less macho. Suddenly, men had their own fashion designers and their own toiletry counters—not to mention the tacit approval of their wives and girlfriends, who had never been particularly pleased with their men's casual, often uncaring attitude toward their own appearance.

Celebrities—*male* celebrities—began to take an active and, what's more, a conspicuous interest in how they looked. Led by athletes (who have always reaped rewards for understanding the correlation between good health and efficient performance) and television personalities (who are well aware of being seen in brutal closeup, night after night, by millions of people), they began not only to use but to endorse products that, only a short time before, no man would admit even knowing about.

Hair driers, moisturizers, body splashes, and bronzers were now out in the open, acceptable not only in one's own medicine cabinet, but in the locker room as well. Men who were accustomed to an occasional splash of cologne soon found that, as often as not, their favorite brand of it had been joined by an after-shave balm, a shampoo, a talc, maybe even a mask. Manufacturers had realized, a little in advance of the rest of us, that men's grooming was potentially very big business indeed. They knew that men who had for some time been in the habit of quietly appropriating a little of the after-sun cream their wife or girlfriend used were now ready for their own supplies. And that all the other men, who'd never dreamed of using anything at all on their faces, weren't far behind.

I don't want to imply that American men had, after years of ignorance, suddenly seen some mystical light and discovered the concept of physical beauty, or turned into a race of narcissists. But they *had*, most definitely, become aware that there were ways they could take care of themselves, upgrade their image (and, with it, their effectiveness) in business as well as in private life, and preserve that commodity so precious to twentieth-century America, youthfulness. The man in the street was learning what we skin-care specialists had known for centuries: that people who take care of their skin look better and don't age as quickly as people who don't take care of it.

Let me stress something right now, at the beginning of what I hope will be a very specific, informative, and persuasive discussion of all aspects of skin care: there is no magic here. Skin care is a matter of effort, knowledge, and application. It is not—I repeat, *not*—a matter of secrets, myths, and celebrity tips. There are some "truths" that are really fallacies: that you should wash your face twice a day with soap; that shaving with the hottest water you can stand is good for you; or that sauna plumps and nourishes the skin. And you'll have to trust me when I tell you not to continue to be the victim of attitudes you learned in childhood, not to do something a certain way simply because you've always done it that way. For underlying my advice you'll always find principles that are solid and based on a knowledge of skin physiology and chemistry.

The word *chemistry* has special meaning for me. I grew up in a small town in Romania and, from earliest boyhood, wanted to be a scientist. I graduated from the University of Cluj with a degree in chemistry and interests that were more medical than aesthetic. Pharmaceutical research into skin care was my first career inclination, and it was only in the course of observing patients' difficulties in dealing—psychologically and emotionally—with the imperfections of their own faces that I came to realize the tremendous importance of cosmetology, of preventive skin care. I began applying my technical knowledge of skin chemistry and physiology to the treatment of the faces of real men and women.

My clinical background and orientation have convinced me of one thing especially: that it's risky to use commercial skin-care products, even the best of which may contain synthetic chemicals and preservatives that are actually toxic. Natural skin-care products are all I use at my clinic, and I make all of them myself. You can do the same, using the simple formulas I'll provide. It takes only a few minutes, right in your own bathroom or kitchen and, in the long run, it's much cheaper than buying them at drug and department stores. Because you make the products yourself, and store them as directed, the concepts of shelf-life and preservatives are irrelevant. You use a product for as long as it lasts, assured of its freshness *without* preservatives. Then you just make a new batch.

I don't want to bore you with my conviction that the natural way is the only sane and sensible way; so much has been written about natural things lately that the word—like *pure* and *organic*—has lost its meaning. But I do want to stress again the dangers of commercial preparations and I think that right now, as we're starting out, is the time to do it.

Obviously, no ethical manufacturer knowingly puts toxic chemicals into his products. The tragedy is that he may not realize he's doing so. Let me give you a very recent example. Substances called emulsifiers are required to hold oil and water—the dual bases of most cosmetic products—together. One of the most common emulsifiers in the industry, used in thousands of such products for more than forty years, is called triethanolamine, or TEA, and it had never given any indication of being anything but safe and non-irritating to the skin. Yet it's recently been discovered, thanks to sophisticated new machinery, that TEA is capable of generating, in certain chemical contexts, significant amounts of a substance called nitrosamine. These nitrosamines can be absorbed through the skin and right into the bloodstream, where, over a period of time, they may have a carcinogenic effect. Ten years ago, nearly all scientists assumed that chemicals used in skin-care products were, considerable evidence notwithstanding, incapable of penetrating the skin at all, so the TEA reversal has had a frightening impact.

I'm not telling the story to alarm you. I'm telling it to make you aware that science is not infallible; that chemicals can be dangerous even when they're believed to be safe; that what you put on your skin matters, and sometimes matters gravely; and that, with such risks to run constantly, natural really *is* better. I'll have more to say on the subject in the formulary in the back of the book. And a great deal to say on a related subject—nutrition, where again natural ingredients are of absolutely fundamental importance—in the chapter I devote to that topic.

You're a man, and you can grow a beard and a mustache, but your skin really is no different, physiologically or chemically, from a woman's. The outermost layer of it may be slightly thicker, but this is the result of more extensive environmental exposure, not some hormonal or biological disparity: the skin has thickened, over the years, to protect itself from sun, wind, cold, and so on. Otherwise, your face is as delicate, sensitive, and excitable as your wife's or girlfriend's. Moreover, you don't wear makeup, as she does, which means you go into the world without even that slim protective margin. You're subject to the whole range of skin ailments and deficiencies: dryness, oiliness, pimples and blackheads, broken capillaries, and premature skin aging. In addition, your skin mirrors inner imbalances, serving as an early-warning system for the body it sheathes, hinting at its secret ailments.

In that sense, it's a direct reflection of your health and state of mind.

Precisely *because* your skin reveals so much about you—how you're feeling, how old you are, what strains and stresses you're under—it's one of the aspects of you that other people notice first. There's no need for them to find it anything less than clear and sanguine, or you anything less than at your peak. Most skin problems can be alleviated, if not completely solved, by adopting the appropriate skin-care routine, taking only a few minutes twice a day. One of the goals of this book is to help you find not only the right products, but also the right procedures.

Because everybody's skin is different and because everybody has different needs, determined by the way he lives and works, you'll find that such a routine is in fact highly individualized, that it involves more than just shaving and keeping your face clean. It's up to you, of course, to decide if good skin is worth ten or twelve minutes a day, plus the cost of a few specialized products (which, as I've promised, you can learn to make yourself). But I have never had a client, male or female, who didn't get a psychological boost from looking better—dramatically better.

I hope that men will soon come to see that how they look is not only important but, with the joint assistance of science and aesthetics, *improvable.* As a specialist in skin care, I hope that they'll be not only interested in taking better care of their skin but become more skilled at doing so. It's my sincere wish that this book—the first ever devoted exclusively to skin care for men—will help them learn how.

MARIO BADESCU'S
SKIN CARE PROGRAM FOR MEN

———•———

ONE

GETTING TO KNOW YOUR FACE

I N THE PREFACE, I had my opportunity to philosophize. Now it's time for me to get down to work. It's time for you to do the same. I hope that you'll read this chapter very carefully. The more you know about the skin—about its structure, functions, and needs—the easier it will be to take care of your own with a minimum of fuss.

BASICS OF SKIN STRUCTURE AND FUNCTION

Your skin is your largest organ, your body's most immediate link with and protection from the outside world. Apart from covering delicate internal organs, its main functions are the regulation of body temperature and the elimination of waste materials through the release of perspiration. It also breathes, absorbing oxygen and expelling carbon dioxide directly, in a sort of autonomous miniature respiration process. This respiration is essential to the skin's own metabolism, which is why so much of skin care revolves around unblocking and increasing the skin's oxygen supply.

The skin consists of two main layers: an outer layer, called the epidermis; and an inner layer, called the dermis. Underlying both is a layer of adipose (or fatty) tissue called the hypodermis.

The epidermis, which is itself constructed of microscopic layers, is designed by nature specifically to withstand the effects of the environment. It is here that dirt from the air in which we spend our lives collects, that wind, sun, and the drying effects of overheated and over air-conditioned rooms take their toll. The epidermis responds to these environmental onslaughts by constantly renewing itself, replacing an entire layer of skin cells with new cells at least once every thirty days. These cells form in the bottom layer of the epidermis and rise through all successive layers, undergoing a growth-maturation-death process called keratinization along the way. By the time they're ready to surface, they are completely keratinized, by which I mean they are quite literally dead, ready to be shed and replaced by a fresh new group of cells. Thus the skin rejuvenates itself. However, although the dead skin cells on the epidermis's surface are quite invisible, they must be constantly and thoroughly cleansed away. Otherwise, the skin takes on a dull, scaly look.

The pores you see in your mirror are actually oil ducts, not sweat ducts as many people think. Since the oil (or sebaceous, in technical language) glands, like the sweat (or sudoriferous) glands, are stimulated by heat, steam baths, saunas, and hot summer weather will temporarily enlarge the pores. When, for one reason or another, these pores become blocked, whiteheads, blackheads, and pimples appear on your skin.

The epidermis also has another important component, a water-attracting compound called the Natural Moisturizing Factor, or NMF, which allows the skin to hydrate itself, to keep itself wet. The amount of NMF in the skin decreases with age, which is one reason why skin tends to get drier as we get older.

All skin problems show up in the epidermis, but the real trouble is often lurking down below, in the dermis, which nourishes the epidermis. The dermis is also the site of the sweat glands, which secrete waste and water; the oil glands, which secrete sebum, a colorless, odorless, oily substance that keeps the skin supple; the hair follicles; the lymph vessels; the nerves and nerve endings; and the blood capillaries that bring oxygen and other indispensable commodities to the skin. This area determines how your skin *looks*.

The dermis is largely made up of a fibrous protein called collagen, which gives the skin its elasticity, providing what we call tone, allowing the skin to stretch, then bounce back again. When this collagen breaks down, as it inevitably does with age, the skin begins to sag. Then wrinkles form. Overexposure to sun and wind causes collagen fibers to break down even faster. To guard against such destruction, a layer of melanin, or pigment cells, lies at the bottom of the epidermis, just above the dermis. The melanin, which is responsible for what we call suntan, is designed to shield the dermis from ultraviolet rays, the kind the sun specializes in. Unfortunately, it is only partially effective. Unlike the epidermis, the dermis does not replace itself; damage occurring within it is irreversible. Worse yet, it tends to be cumulative.

Below the dermis is the layer of fatty connective tissue I mentioned above, called the hypodermis. The hypodermis is like a big cushion. It protects the dermis, and is responsible for supporting and contouring, or rounding out, the skin. (The hypodermis is practically nonexistent around the eyes, part of the reason why this is such a delicate area, and so quick to age.) Crash diets often cause too much fatty tissue to be lost, resulting in sags and a general loss of contour. This can be avoided through proper nutrition, however, as you'll see later on in this book.

That, in short, is how the skin is structured. Let's begin now to see how it *works*.

THE pH FACTOR

I've never understood why this simple concept has aroused so much confusion and misunderstanding; perhaps it's the abbreviation itself that's the problem. The pH factor refers, simply, to hydrogen potential, which is to say, to the balance of hydrogen ions in a given substance. It tells us if the substance is acid, alkaline, or neutral, and is measured on a scale of zero to fourteen. Seven is a neutral pH, anything below seven is acid, and anything above, alkaline. The normal "resting" pH of the skin is just about 5.5, which means it is slightly acid. This acidity is the result of secretions by the oil and sweat glands, which combine on the surface of the skin to form what is known as the acid mantle.

The acid mantle is your skin's armor, its sole protection against the environment. As such, it must be stimulated, encouraged, and appreciated. Only two things can destroy the acid mantle: illness and alkaline soaps. Both will upset the pH balance, making the skin veer either toward excess acidity or excess alkalinity, with results ranging from acne to extreme and uncomfortable dryness.

Although the inadvisability of using alkaline products on the skin has been common knowledge for thirty years or so, the pH factor first began to attract the attention of the media about ten years ago. Since then, many products with acid or neutral pH's have become widely available. The fact that a product is acid, however, does *not* mean it won't remove your skin's acid mantle. The acid mantle is composed of water- and fat-soluble substances that even the gentlest cleanser can strip away. Only an extremely well-balanced cleanser can maintain the acid mantle *and* remove dirt at the same time. One thing you can be thankful for: When it comes to the pH factor, men are luckier than women, in that, except for actors and models, they do not wear makeup. No cleanser can remove makeup without removing the acid mantle as well.

Maintaining the correct pH is of most significance to those two extremes of skin type, acne and aging skin. In the case of acne, excessive, disordered glandular secretions make the skin's pH go haywire, sometimes changing from acid to alkaline and back again in a single day. In aging skin, glandular secretions slow to a trickle; there may be little if anything left of the acid mantle.

Don't let all this intimidate you, though. I've thought through the technical aspects of acidity vs. alkalinity, which means you don't have to. Simply by using the products and techniques recommended in the chapter on your particular skin type, you will be able to balance, maintain, and correct your skin's pH. As I stated in my introduction, there are no impenetrable mysteries connected with skin care.

SKIN TYPES

Knowing your skin and its needs is the single most important prerequisite for taking effective care of it, yet few of the people (and an especially low percentage of the men) who come to my clinic for the first time know the first thing about their skin. Only by understanding your skin *type* can you have any idea how to help or correct the skin itself. Moreover, skin type can change with the seasons as well as the years, and each individual skin type has its own idiosyncrasies, its own ways of misbehaving and falling short.

Basically, there are three types of skin: normal, oily, and dry.

Normal skin is healthy, balanced skin. The oil glands secrete enough sebum to lock moisture onto the skin's surface, but not so much as to clog the pores. The dermis sends plenty of blood to the surface, while the epidermis is thin and smooth enough to let an even, rosy color show through. In short, all the factors we have discussed in the preceding paragraphs are in perfect equilibrium.

Once every month or so, I'll see a man with normal skin. His pores will be barely visible, and they'll be uniform in size.

He will have no blackheads or other blemishes, and only a few tiny lines in the eye area, regardless of his age. As a rule, I don't see men (or women either) over age twenty-five with normal skin. If you're lucky and are one of the rare exceptions, your skin-care routine will be a matter of maintenance, rather than correction. But your maintenance routine is just as important as that of the man with problem skin, and you must abide by it. Even the healthiest complexion can easily be destroyed through improper or insufficient care.

Oily skin is caused by oversecretion of the oil glands. This situation does not, in itself, make for an unhealthy complexion. On the contrary, oily skin is less prone to aging and wrinkling than other skin types, since the abundance of oil helps keep precious moisture from evaporating from the epidermis. On the other hand, clogged pores and blackheads are perennial problems for oily-skinned people, and care is needed to keep dead skin cells from sticking together and piling up in layers on the skin's surface. Oily skin is thick, with large pores clearly visible everywhere except around the eyes and neck. It is often sallow and rough-textured.

Dry skin, the opposite of oily skin, occurs when the oil glands don't produce sufficient oil to lubricate the skin properly. Dry skin is thin and often flaky, with virtually invisible pores. It is likely to have many fine wrinkles. And it tends to be easily irritated.

So far, it's relatively simple. But skin analysis and skin care are complicated by the existence of two *sub*-categories—dehydrated skin and combination skin—and by the fact that most of us have skin that is not always just one type.

Dehydrated skin, which is often confused with dry skin for obvious reasons, is in fact the result not of lack of oil, but of loss of moisture; the skin is, to a greater or lesser degree, dying of thirst. This water loss can be caused by any number of factors: exposure to sun and wind; lack of humidity; glandular malfunction or hormonal imbalance; crash diets that work by dehydrating the body; or just plain age, with its accompanying slowdown in the production of NMF. Dehydrated skin is very common. Its signature is a network of fine wrinkles, particularly around the eyes and cheeks. Dehydrated areas will usually be dry to the touch, dull in color, flat in texture, and clearly lacking in elasticity. What most people don't realize, and what causes a lot of mistakes in skin-care routines, is that both oily *and* dry skins can suffer from dehydration.

Combination skin is just what its name implies: a combination of dry, oily, or normal areas, all on the same face. A man with combination skin (80 percent of all men have it) is usually dry around the cheeks, eyes, and neck, while oily in the area we call the T-zone, the vertical bar from chin to nose and up to the forehead. Combination skin takes a bit more effort if it is to be cared for completely, since each area makes its own separate demands. But once you have perfected your routine, it will be necessary to spend only a few extra minutes in return for consistently healthy, trouble-free skin all over your face.

Now let's look at you, and analyze *your* particular skin type. This shouldn't take more than a quarter of an hour, but I urge you to be precise and careful in your analysis. Let me say right now that I do not think you should waste time just worrying about your skin. Staring for hours at a pimple, a broken capillary, or a wrinkle won't make it go away; a second is all it takes to see that the problem is there and that something should be done about it. You should be conscious, however, of the overall surface of your skin and the ways in which it changes, from facial area to facial area and, for that matter, from April to August to November. Check your analysis every month or so, or whenever you notice any striking differences that might arise from environmental factors, or from the use of new skin-care products.

As your skin changes, you should also expect to have to alter your products slightly. A man with extremely oily skin, for instance, should start out using a relatively strong cleansing lotion (we will get to them in a moment). As his skin improves, he'll wish to decrease the strength of the lotion to make it more appropriate to his more normal skin. Obviously, the state and type of your skin determine the products you use, and a change in any one of the product categories may necessitate changes in the others.

DETERMINING YOUR SKIN TYPE
The Cigarette-Paper Test

The simplest way to test your skin type is with a few pieces of plain white cigarette paper and a strongly, even unflatteringly lit mirror. First, wash your face—not with soap, but with an ordinary, drugstore-variety bland, unmentholated shaving cream. Then wait the two or three hours necessary for your skin to regain its natural acid mantle. Yes, it really takes that long.

Now, press a piece of plain white cigarette paper firmly on one section of your face. Leave it there for a few seconds. If the paper adheres to the face and shows an oily spot when held up to the light, you have oily skin. If the paper doesn't stick and shows no spot, you have dry or dehydrated skin.

If the paper does stick to the face but shows no oily spots when you remove it, you have normal skin.

Test all areas of the face separately. If the paper shows oiliness in some areas, dryness in others, you have combination skin.

On a hot day, a spot on the paper may simply be perspiration. Wait a few seconds, then check the paper again; perspiration will have evaporated, whereas an oil spot will remain. Don't use the paper test on the eye area; this is dry for everybody, no matter what his skin type. Likewise, most people have relatively dry skin on the neck, and skin that is at least slightly oily on and around the nose. The cheeks, the forehead, and the chin are more likely to reveal the true condition of your skin, in all its various aspects.

Use your mirror and the descriptions of skin types I have already provided to corroborate the paper test's findings. Now you should have a good idea of your skin type. Later, I'll discuss every skin type—its needs, aberrations, and product requirements—in detail. Before I do that, I want to give you a general idea of the *range* of products you may be dealing with.

THE KINDS OF PRODUCTS YOU'LL USE

All skin-care products do at least one of five things:

1. *Deep cleanse,* since skin can't function properly if dirt, cellular wastes, and toxins are not removed thoroughly on a day-to-day basis.
2. *Correct skin conditions* that exist but can be remedied, such as dryness, oiliness, sensitivity, and acne.
3. *Stimulate,* by boosting local metabolism, especially where it's fallen off as the result of age.
4. *Maintain* the skin's suppleness, tone, and elasticity.
5. *Protect* skin from the ravages of the environment.

On a short-term basis, these preparations will relieve dryness, oiliness, and irritability, as well as prevent the formation of wrinkles. Long-term use, over months and years, will endow the skin with a smooth, healthy texture, with suppleness and strength. Since the skin will always be moisturized, not only will superficial wrinkles not form, but the onset of deeper wrinkles and expression lines will be postponed by a good ten years, and sometimes by as many as twenty-five. Nor, if the knowledge and the products are available to him, is there any reason for a man in his teens and twenties to suffer pits and pockmarks. All of this is unnecessary and debilitating.

All that said by way of prelude, I want you to prepare yourself for a shock.

I do not sell soap in my clinic. Men, especially, are confused by this at first. "But how can I get my face clean if I don't use soap?" they ask.

The fact is that soap certainly won't get your face clean. What it will do is encourage wrinkles and aggravating pimples, blackheads, and rashes.

Most soaps are strongly alkaline. As you'll remember from our talk about the pH factor, any alkaline product destroys the skin's protective acid mantle. Soap also strips off natural oils, and carries away the water-soluble NMF, leaving your skin vulnerable to aging and wrinkling—*unnecessary* aging and wrinkling. Since soap is one of the strong emulsifiers, it can easily irritate your skin, which is probably already sensitive from a lifetime of shaving. Finally, soap is impervious to rinsing. No matter how much you try, it will leave an invisible residue on the skin, dulling its luster, neutralizing its acidity, and binding itself to natural skin proteins, where it exerts a dehydrating, denaturing power.

Now this sounds so dangerous you might think your skin would be ruined forever after using soap even once, which of course isn't the case at all. The damage is, rather, slow and cumulative. My clients are always amazed at how quickly their skin improves, both in looks and in texture, when they switch from soap to the gentler kind of cleanser I recommend, namely cleansing lotions.

Cleansing Lotions: A cleansing lotion contains, depending on skin type, varying degrees of witch hazel, rose water, alcohol, honey or a related form of fructose or glucose, and possibly a fruit, vegetable, or herbal extract. The cleansing action comes mainly from the essential oils in the plant extracts, which dissolve dirt, and from the alcohol. This alcohol must be very carefully balanced, since too high an alcohol content can have a dehydrating effect. (Many alcohol-based lotions, cleansers, toners, and astringents contain between 50 and 80 percent alcohol, which is much too high. The ones I recommend are adjusted to contain between 5 and 30 percent.) These cleansing lotions are mildly antiseptic and toning; they encourage, rather than erode, the acid mantle and aid natural hydration. By thoroughly but gently removing dirt and pollutants, they allow the skin to do what it really wants to do anyway—function efficiently. In addition, men's cleansing lotions also contain agents to reduce irritation and swelling, and to promote healing of all the microabrasions inevitably acquired in shaving.

Before/After Shave Moisturizer: This product has a dual function: to soften and lubricate the beard prior to blade shaving, and to protect, soothe, and hydrate skin afterwards.

After-Shave Mask: This is a mineral-based product applied to the face after shaving to counteract severe irritation. It should not be used daily, unless absolutely necessary, if only because of the inconvenience inherent in its five- to twenty-minute application time. But it is a very handy thing to have at your disposal if you tend to get rashes and pimples in the beard area.

At-Home Masks: These are simple products, related to the After-Shave Mask, again requiring applications of up to twenty minutes two or three times a week. They vary according to skin type, and they serve a variety of purposes, depending on their ingredient mix. Regular use will boost skin metabolism and eliminate dead cells that can prevent skin from functioning at its peak. The at-home masks have a hydrating and firming action that helps eliminate superficial lines and maintains a good moisture balance. Depending on your skin type and their formulation, they can work to stimulate or to control the oil glands. They'll also aid in removing blackheads and healing pimples.

Superficial Peelings: Made from a paste of water and wheat bran or cornmeal, the superficial peeling is rubbed briskly into the skin to remove part of the layer of dead cells on the skin surface. These cells obstruct respiration of the deeper skin layers and make the skin dull and unhealthy looking. Peelings also help to remove superficial blackheads.

Many commercial peelings are made, but I can't recommend most of them. They come in two varieties. First, there are the so-called scrub creams, which usually contain an enzyme or caustic chemical, plus a powder abrasive. These can be harmful to the skin, causing irritation, dehydration, and broken capillaries.

Second are the polyester web sponges recommended by many dermatologists for superficial peeling. These are more closely related to cornmeal and wheat bran peels because their action is mechanical rather than chemical. But they are dangerous. I do not exaggerate when I say that I've had thousands of people who, after using these sponges improperly, came into my clinic with irritation, pimples, scars, and irremediable damage to the surface capillaries. I have no doubt sponges can be of great value when they are used correctly, but I don't see many people who do use them correctly. In the meantime, there are easier and safer methods.

Even my superficial peelings are to be considered a special measure, not to be employed every day; in fact no more than once a week, and sometimes as infrequently as once a month.

Cream Emulsions: These are combinations of rich oils, plus water and water-retaining ingredients. Their purpose is to replace oil and water lacking in dry skin, as well as to stimulate oil-gland secretion whenever possible. There are two kinds of cream emulsion—eye creams and night creams, the latter to be used only for dry or aging skin.

Every man or woman over the age of twenty-one should apply an eye cream in the morning and in the evening, as part of the daily cleansing routine. There are no exceptions. The critical areas are just under the eyes and from lid to eyebrow. The skin here is extremely thin and fragile, lacking oil, water, and any significant elastic tissue support. It is, as a result, extremely vulnerable to dehydration, wrinkles, and sagging. A few lines around the eye are inevitable, of course, since you can't—and wouldn't want to—avoid the little creases that come from years of smiling. However, assiduous lubrication and hydration can keep such lines to a minimum. Eye creams are thick and rich—they have to be if they're going to be effective. Don't worry about visibility; a minute after application, you blot off the residue with a tissue, leaving only an invisible protective film.

Don't underestimate the importance of eye creams in your daily routine. I repeat that this is the most fragile area of your face and the one most prone to external damage. It must be protected at all times, especially by men who work or play outdoors.

Night creams are less rich than eye creams. They are meant to be applied to the entire face and neck after the nightly cleansing, but they should be used only by men with very dry or aging skin. They would, quite frankly, clog the pores of an oily skin. Even in the case of the driest type of skin, they should be used only every other night. Why? Because you don't want your skin to become addicted to them. The oil glands, you see, can sense the presence of oil on the skin, and when they do, they decrease production of their own precious oil. Yet without extra help, the glands may not function properly either. Caught in this bind, you have no choice but to apply night cream on alternate nights. This ensures maximum activity on the part of the oil glands by keeping them stimulated.

A NOTE ON BASIC APPLICATION TECHNIQUES

Although the products you use vary with your skin type and seasonal needs, the basic techniques you'll use to apply them remain unvarying and, you'll be happy to hear, uncomplicated. Not only does proper application ensure a product's effectiveness, but it gives you the added benefits of a once-over-lightly massage, relaxed muscles, improved circulation, and a smoothing of the facial contours. We'll talk about a full-scale facial massage in another chapter, but in the meantime you should familiarize yourself with the following basic principles of product application. They pertain most obviously to creams and other substances applied with your fingertips, but they can be adapted to lotions, which should be applied with balls of cotton.

First, using both hands at once, one on each side of the face, smooth a cream *upward* and *outward* from chin to ears, nose to temples, and up between the eyes, over the forehead to the temples. The upward and outward motion is very important, because that's really how your skin is draped over the muscles of your face. To do anything else is to tug at the skin, stretching it needlessly and threatening its elasticity. Likewise, when you apply a cream to your throat—which you should do because your skin can get very dry down there—first tilt your head up a little, then, holding all four fingers together, massage slightly with long sweeping strokes, again *upward* and *outward*. One extra detail here: use the left hand on the right side of the throat and vice versa, alternating left and right strokes.

As for the nose itself, apply a minimum number of preparations to it because it is so well endowed with its own oil glands. Massage the area around the nose, though, using small circles and the middle finger of each hand.

The eyes, delicate as they are, require a degree of special handling. Never rub or stroke here. Rather, pat gently with your fingertips over the eyelids from inner corner to outer. Repeat the inner-to-outer movement, again using a series of pats, on the superdelicate under-eye area.

This is the most basic, across-the-board information I can provide on skin care. Obviously, I haven't begun to deal with special problems or needs, or even prescribed programs for the various skin types. The next two chapters will be devoted to precisely that, however. I suggest that you read very, very closely the material dealing with *your* skin type, followed by the chapter on regimens and techniques; then turn to the formulary in the back of the book to learn the composition of the products I've prescribed for you. Of course you'll also want to read chapters dealing with any skin disorder that you may have—say, acne or premature aging. And I must insist that, as soon as you've done all this, you turn to the chapter on nutrition. It's extremely important, for you must treat your skin from the *inside* as well as the outside.

·

TWO

ALL ABOUT SKIN TYPES

IF YOU PERFORMED the cigarette-paper test described in the last chapter, you know what your skin type is. But you don't yet know all that you should about it. This chapter will tell you. By all means, read the whole chapter. But if you're pressed for time—or simply are anxious to get going with your own individualized regimen—you may want to read only the section dealing with your own skin type, whether it's dry/dehydrated, oily, or normal/combination.

DRY AND DEHYDRATED SKIN

As you'll recall, dry and dehydrated are two different—but easily confused—skin classifications. Dry skin is the opposite of oily skin, and occurs whenever the oil glands are too lazy or tired to lubricate the skin properly. Dry skin—thin and tiny-pored, often flaky or possessed of many fine wrinkles—is the more serious condition. Dry skin is frequently sensitive and easily irritated. Older people are more likely to suffer from it than teen-agers; in fact, almost everybody's skin becomes drier as he ages.

While dry skin results from a lack of oil, dehydrated skin is caused by the loss of moisture; dehydrated skin simply can't absorb and retain enough water to keep itself vital and supple. You can recognize dehydrated skin by its parchment-like texture, its thinness, its lack of elasticity. If you pinch a small section of skin away from your cheekbone and it fails to bounce back almost faster than your eye can follow it, chances are your skin is dehydrated. (Dry skin is usually more supple and *will* bounce back.) Dehydrated skin is identified by a network of fine wrinkles, particularly around the eyes and cheeks. Often there are broken capillaries close to the skin's surface, too. All these symptoms point to the skin's unhealthily low water level. Dehydrated skin is more often the result of environmental factors—especially steam heat and air-conditioning—than biological ones, although, as we'll see, what's going on *inside* your body can cause dehydrated skin, as well.

Causes of Dry and Dehydrated Skin

As I've already pointed out, dry skin is often simply a legacy of the aging process, like the deceleration of metabolism or the need for less sleep. Dry skin can also come about through malfunctioning of the endocrine glands (or other hormonal imbalances), or through inadequate diet, most commonly a diet that is too low in oils and fats. Like oily skin, however, it is first and foremost genetically determined, a matter of what you inherited at birth.

Dehydrated skin sometimes results from the same range of glandular malfunctions as dry skin, as well as from the kind of quick weight-loss diets that work by dehydrating the body—and with it the skin. Most typically, though, dehydrated skin results from how you live. That is, if you spend enough time in the sun or the wind or the cold your skin will become naturally dehydrated. Nor are overheated or over air-conditioned offices and homes any better for the skin. In both such cases, room humidity is so low that it actually drains moisture from the skin. A humidifier, at least for your bedroom or perhaps in your office, would aid greatly in combatting this peculiarly modern skin problem.

Pros and Cons of Dry Skin

Dry skin, besides being a simple reflection of the aging process, will also—in true vicious-circle style—itself age faster than oily skin. (Oily skin is, after all, both lubricated and protected by that film of oil.) As I have previously noted, dry skin is especially likely to be plagued by many fine lines and broken capillaries. And it can become sensitive, even irritated, again because it is so vulnerable, so unprotected. Finally, it falls prey to dehydration much more frequently than oily or normal skin, thereby putting a double strain on the complexion.

What's good about dry skin? Very little, really, which is why we'll be setting out to correct it, to make it function as normally as possible. But if you'd like to look on the bright side of things, it's true that dry skin is less likely than oily skin to develop most kinds of blemishes—blackheads, pimples, and acne of all kinds. It may not be totally immune to such problems (it is, after all, filled with pores, even if those pores are largely invisible), but it generally isn't at their mercy. Moreover, the texture is more attractive than that of oily skin. Is there any redeeming virtue to having dehydrated skin? None at all. Luckily, however, we can *de*-dehydrate it.

Taking Care of Your Dry and Dehydrated Skin

Believe it or not, you probably already are taking care of it, at least a little. Every time you shave, you're stimulating the beard region of your face, boosting the supply of oxygen to the skin, increasing the circulation of the blood, and generally upping the level of all skin functions, including the production of that vital oil. In general our aim will be to encourage your whole face—and not just the beard area—to produce more oil. Or, in the case of dehydrated skin, to absorb and retain more water. The program of cleansing and treatment that I'll be recommending in the following chapters applies to both skins, and makes use of identical preparations. (In some circumstances, however, dehydrated skin requires extra moisturizing, which I'll note as we go along.)

Your routine consists of two phases, a morning one and a bedtime one. They are similar, really, both designed to stimulate the oil glands and lubricate the face, as well as to cleanse and tone it, but the bedtime phase is just a little more elaborate. It's during the night, you see, that your skin, just like the rest of you, renews itself, and the way must be carefully paved for this renewal process. Of course, as I explained in Chapter I, you'll *never* use soap to cleanse your skin. Neither, for that matter, will soap be used for any other skin type, but in your case it's especially critical to avoid it, because of its drying nature. Your skin is already too dry!

OILY SKIN

If the paper adhered to your skin in the cigarette-paper test, showing oily spots in most areas of the face, especially on the forehead, cheeks, chin, and nose, you have an oily skin. Even so, the eye area (from just below the brow to just under the eyes) and the neck area will probably show up as dry while the area around the sides of the cheeks, just by the ears, frequently shows up as dehydrated, no matter what your skin type.

You'll recognize oily skin by its large, visible pores and generally coarse, rough texture. An oily skin is also thicker than a dry skin. Some of the skin pores may be even more enlarged because they are clogged with oil-gland secretions. Blackheads can appear anywhere on the skin, especially around the nose and lip areas. (Blackheads are hard plugs of oil that turn black when they *oxidize* upon coming in contact with the air.)

Causes of Oily Skin

Oily skin is caused by over-activity of the oil glands beneath the skin. This is often genetic. An oily skin actually has more oil glands than a dry skin, and this abundance of oil glands is one of the things that give an oily skin its extra thickness. However, excessive oiliness can also be caused by a number of dietary factors, especially by a lack of any of the B-complex vitamins. Many men with oily skin find it has a tendency to develop into a light or heavy acne condition; often this can be controlled by sticking to a high fiber diet. This information is covered in detail in the nutrition chapter.

Pros and Cons of Oily Skin

An oily skin tends to be less dehydrated than a dry skin. This is because that film of oil on the skin's surface helps to lock in moisture. And since lack of moisture is the primary cause of superficial wrinkles, men with oily skin tend to look younger than men with dry skin. Their skin will also stay supple longer. The only catch is that since an oily skin is thicker than a dry skin, the wrinkles you do have will be deeper than those on a dry skin.

Thickness gives oily skin one of its biggest advantages because the tiny blood vessels, the capillaries, are much farther away from the surface. This means that oily skin isn't as subject to broken capillaries, which are visible as small, thin, red or purplish veins, just under the surface of the skin.

Those heavy oil secretions can, however, cause some problems. These will vary in importance with each individual case, and can change according to the season (since the skin produces even more oil in hot weather). But oily skin problems can easily be controlled and corrected by your daily skin program. The main trouble with excess oil is that it becomes mixed with dead skin cells, dirt, and environmental pollutants on the skin surface. This creates a stubborn film that is a perfect breeding ground for pimples and blackheads. What's more, the layer of oil can give a sallow, unhealthy appearance to your skin. It also prevents oxygen from being absorbed by the skin and carbon dioxide from being eliminated from it. This is important because fully 3 percent of the body's respiration occurs directly through the skin; when the skin can't breathe through this oily film, it begins to look dead. The oily film also makes the face look shiny, of course, which, in excess, is not particularly attractive either. A healthy face should glow from its high moisture content and its healthy blood flow, not from excess oil.

Taking Care of Your Oily Skin

The main objective of your daily skin routine will be to calm down those oil glands, gradually discouraging them from producing excess oil while maintaining just enough to keep your skin properly lubricated, supple, and healthy looking. Proper cleansing will also keep your pores unclogged, discouraging breakouts and allowing your skin to breathe. Within a few months, your pores will become less visible and your skin's texture will become finer. Moreover, once you've begun hydrating your skin properly, the superficial wrinkles that may have formed around your eyes and on your neck will start to diminish.

Don't worry. You're not going to have to spend hours caring for your face every day. If anything, this routine will probably reduce the amount of fussing you do over your skin, since one of the big problems with oily skin is that it encourages its owner to over-cleanse. If you, like so many men, have been scrubbing away at your face with harsh soaps and astringents several times a day in an effort to battle an apparently never-ending gush of oil, you can stop right now. Not only do those products and all that scrubbing ultimately dry the outer layer of your skin, so that you end up having to deal with the problems of both dehydrated *and* oily skin, but, by totally stripping your skin of oils, they actually encourage your oil glands to work that much harder. The oil glands are, in your case, overzealous to begin with; as soon as they sense that your skin surface is unprotected, they start pumping out oil for all they're worth. I'll explain this in greater detail later on in this chapter.

No, what I advise you to do is limit your routine to a proper cleansing twice a day, using a thorough but gentle lotion cleanser you can make yourself at home quite inexpensively, from safe, natural products. I also suggest you get into the habit of lubricating those areas of your skin that need it; that's right, even oily skin needs help in spots, especially in the area around the eyes, since absolutely no one produces enough oil to safeguard that delicate tissue. And if you have dry spots elsewhere on your face, as many oily skins do, you'll begin to take proper care of those, too, with an easy-to-use moisturizer. All of this will boil down into the two simple daily routines, one in the morning and one at night, that I've already referred to.

NORMAL AND COMBINATION SKIN

Normal Skin

Normal skin is the rarest complexion type of all; as I have already noted, I almost never see anybody—man *or* woman— over the age of twenty-five who has normal skin. You may argue, of course, that people with normal skin don't need to see a skin-care expert in the first place. That may be the case. But let me assure you, even on the street, in restaurants, at the theater I see very little skin that can be considered normal.

What *is* normal skin? Well, it's healthy skin, skin that

exists in a perfect equilibrium between oiliness on the one hand and dryness on the other, that has a balanced pH factor, and that is smooth and satiny in texture. A magnifying mirror would reveal that all the pores, regardless of their position on the face, are of roughly the same size, not large, just barely visible, yet noticeably less taut and tiny than the shrunken pores of a dry skin. If you pull a section of normal skin with your fingers, it will bounce back with elasticity. The dermis sends plenty of blood to the surface, while the epidermis is thin enough to let an even, rosy color show through. Finally, there are no visible blackheads or other blemishes, and though there may be a few lines around the eyes and the sides of the nose, they are what I'd call expression lines rather than wrinkles.

Combination Skin

Combination skin, by contrast, is the type I encounter most frequently. It's so common, it would seem to have become the norm, but the skin itself is anything but the normal skin I described above. Rather, it is characterized by oiliness in some areas, generally the chin, nose, and forehead (the so-called "T-zone"), with all the standard features of oiliness— shininess, enlarged pores, even blackheads. Other areas, most notably the cheeks, neck, sides of the jaw, and around the eyes, will be dry, normal, or dehydrated. *They* may manifest such typical dry-skin traits as tautness, loss of elasticity, flakiness, or wrinkling.

I estimate that at least 80 percent of the men whose skin I examine have combination skin. Taking care of combination skin can be tricky and, in a way, require a higher degree of individualized attention than taking care of any other type, since each area makes its own demands, but unless your combination skin is excessively oily in the T zone, or excessively dry in other areas, you can maintain it by following what is pretty much the regimen of a person with normal skin. In just a minute, I'll be showing you how. And I'll stress the two exceptions to a normal skin-care regimen that you'll have to make.

Does it seem strange to you that the least common skin type (at least among adults)—normal—and the most common—combination—should be treated in the same chapter? They are being grouped together because neither is a truly *extreme* skin type. Normal skin is, by definition, healthy, out of danger (but still requiring maintenance if it is to be preserved), well balanced. And even combination skin tends not to be as oily in the T-zone as *truly* oily skin is, as dry in the cheeks, neck, and eye areas as *truly* dry skin is. It may not be balanced, exactly, but its excesses are, more often than not, easily enough controlled. With the proper degree of attention, of course.

Let me conclude with a special plea to any reader lucky enough to have, whatever his age, skin that is normal. Please, follow my instructions carefully. I want you to *keep* this great, cooperative skin you were born with and have been lucky enough to hang onto past puberty. I know it seems to require a minimum of care, but it's not indestructible. You really have to be vigilant if it's going to stay healthy and balanced.

Taking Care of Your Normal Skin

Your daily routine will revolve around keeping your skin cleansed and nourished. In addition, you should give yourself a facial treatment once a month or so (see next chapter) to *deep*-cleanse the complexion and to stimulate those already well-behaved inner layers. After all, you want that spirit of cooperation to go on.

When you want to look particularly good, you can use a mask. I'll provide a description of the most basic kind (I call it the after-shave mask) as well as of some other, more specialized, even rarefied ones. A mask makes your skin glow; it also tightens it, and counteracts any tendency you might have toward blotchiness or congestion.

Taking Care of Your Combination Skin

In general, a combination skin is treated in the same manner as a normal one. Of course, if it is very, very oily in the T-zone or very, very dry in the other areas, it will have to be treated in those places as if it were oily or dry skin. That means that, unfortunately, you'll need to make two kinds of cleansing lotions, two kinds of before/after shave moisturizer—two sets of everything but shaving cream and eye cream, in fact. However, in the majority of cases, such extreme measures aren't necessary. All you have to remember are the following two points:

(1) Don't apply before/after shave emulsion or night cream to the T-zone area; this would only intensify the oiliness.

(2) When you give yourself a mask, either alone or as part of the full facial, you must treat the two different skin types of your face with two different masks. In the formulary, I try to make this as easy as possible for you by providing a double mask that makes use of a common ingredient—powdered brewer's yeast.

THREE

DAILY REGIMENS
AND SPECIAL TREATMENTS

YOUR DAILY skin-care regimen—no matter what your skin type is—consists of two treatments, one to be carried out when you get up in the morning and one before you go to bed at night. Each treatment is predicated on the same principles, those of cleansing, toning, and lubricating the skin, but the bedtime treatment is just a little bit amplified. As I've said before, it's during the night that your skin, just like the rest of you, renews itself, and the way must be carefully paved for this renewal process. In addition, there are special procedures you ought to be familiar with, which can be used from two or three times a week to once a month or so, depending on your own schedule, temperament, and needs. These are meant to provide special nourishment or extra-deep cleansing for the complexion. They're as much a part of your overall skin-care regimen as what you do every morning and evening, and I'll describe them in detail at the end of the chapter.

Needless to say, all the products I describe, from cleansing lotion to rich facial masks, can easily be made at home, using simple, natural products, and for a great deal less money than you're probably spending right now. (You'll find them listed, with ingredients and instructions, in the formulary section in the back of the book.) Most important, you'll ensure the purity of your preparations. If *you*'ve made them, they can't be adulterated and they don't have to contain the preservatives necessary for the long shelf-life they would have to have in a drug or department store.

MORNING TREATMENT

Everybody's in a hurry in the morning. You have to shave, of course, and I suggest that you begin there. You'll cleanse and tone your face in one step—never with soap, as I've mentioned before, but with a non-drying, specially formulated cleansing lotion. Then you'll moisturize. All told, it shouldn't take much longer than your present morning program of shaving and washing with soap and water. And you rest secure in the knowledge that with this bare minimum of steps, you're establishing and eventually preserving the health of your skin. The only equipment you'll need is a towel and some cotton balls or pieces of cotton, available in every supermarket and drugstore. All-cotton balls, by the way, are superior to the polyester ones, which can sometimes cause allergies.

Here, step by step, is your program:

(1) Shave. There's a whole chapter on this subject coming up, and I know that you'll want to read it closely; shaving is, after all, a fact of daily life, and one that can be problematical. In the meantime, I do want to say that you're free, in the case of shaving cream, to go on using any commercial product that you're accustomed to, provided it's fragrance-free. Shaving creams, as a general rule, are very safe, reliable, and efficiently packaged, and there are even special ones, containing lanolin, for dry skin. However, if you *do* want to make your own shaving cream, it *will* be less expensive. (I provide a formula for it.)

(2) Apply cleansing lotion. Moisten, but don't saturate, a cotton ball with lotion and gently stroke over the entire sur-

face of the face and neck with upward and outward motions. Repeat with fresh applications of lotion on fresh cotton until the cotton no longer picks up any traces of dirt. The recipe for the cleansing lotion that you'll use is formulated with your specific skin type in mind, and appears in the formulary in this book.

(3) Rinse your face and neck with lukewarm tap water. This is an optional step, but you will enjoy incorporating it into your morning routine. After all, a splash of water on the face is refreshing. And water wasn't at fault in the old face-washing habit you practiced for so many years; it was soap. After your splash, blot completely dry with a towel. Don't rub too hard or stretch out the skin. In fact, if you leave a little moisture on the skin, you'll be one step ahead, for now is the time that you'll lock the moisture in by hydrating your face.

A special word to men with oily skin: some of you are given to scalding your faces with gallons of *hot* water, in the misguided belief that this is the only way to get your skin clean. This is totally unnecessary; if you've used your cleansing lotion properly, it's already clean. Besides, hot water actually stimulates those overactive sebaceous glands of yours. So stick with the *lukewarm* splash I recommend.

(4) Apply eye cream. Let me say it again: everybody, man or woman, over the age of twenty-one, regardless of skin type, needs an eye cream. (Even that rare complexion, the normal skin, has no protection, no inherent balance, in the area around the eye.) The eye area must be lubricated regularly and often if it's not to begin wrinkling and sagging. Your eye cream (see the formulary and note that eye cream is one thing that doesn't vary according to skin type) will be a little on the heavy side—just as it should be, considering how rich it is in lubricating and hydrating ingredients. To apply, dab some cream under each eye and gently massage over the lid

and under-eye crescent, working from the outer corner in *under the eye*, then from the inner corner out *across the lid.* Blot off any excess with a tissue. Be very, very careful never to stretch the skin of the eye area; it's super-delicate.

(5) Apply before/after shave moisturizer. Moisturizers lubricate the skin, by sealing in moisture, and are a critical link in the good skin-care chain; moreover, the moisturizers I will teach you to make contain other soothing and healing ingredients. To apply, take a dab on your fingertips—not too much, though: this is another case of "less is more." Apply a thin layer over your entire face, even *over* the eye cream. Apply to your neck (where, as you'll recall, there are few oil glands), too, using gentle upward strokes.

You noticed the name *before*/after shave moisturizer? Yes, you can also use this product *before* shaving to soothe and protect the skin, prevent dehydration and overcleansing from the application of shaving cream, and help avoid rashes, razor burns, and the hundreds of microabrasions that occur as a result of shaving. Simply apply to the beard area *after* you've moistened it but before applying shaving cream if shaving is a problematic and painful procedure for you. This is strictly an optional step.

A note on the seasonal use of moisturizer: In the winter, many men will wish to switch from their regular before/after shave moisturizer (which, with a high water content, can actually freeze on the face in extremely cold weather) to a light protective cream, which you'll find a formula for in the section for your skin type in the formulary. When you use a protective cream, be sure to blot off any excess with a tissue; in the case of the moisturizer, blotting is out of place, as the stuff must *remain* on the skin if it's to do any good.

A special note to men with oily skin: your attitude to moisturizers must be one of relative caution. Unlike

men who have dry or normal skin, yours is already over-lu-
bricating itself without any help from you. You'll still want to
use the before/after shave moisturizer as a pre-shave condi-
tioner, especially if you traditionally have problems with the
shaving process. Oily skin doesn't mean that skin can't be
sensitive, too. And in the winter, it will give you extra protection against dehydration. But use it sparingly, only on the
part of the face you shave and on any conspicuously dry
patches. In the summer, when heat further stimulates your
hyperactive sebaceous glands, your cleansing lotion should
give you all the daily protection you need, unless there are
dry patches on your face—around the cheekbones, for instance—or unless you've been exposed to sun and wind.
Then use the moisturizer, just as men with dry skin do.

That's the total morning program. It may seem like a lot right
now, but I assure you, it takes little more time to do it than it
does to read about it. You may not be accustomed to the idea
of using an eye cream and a moisturizer or, for that matter, of
living without soaps and astringents, but once you see how
quickly and how dramatically the tone and texture of your
skin improve, I'm sure you'll have no difficulty in changing
your old habits for new and better ones. Dry-skinned men,
especially, will wonder how they ever got by without the lubrication afforded by a moisturizer.

JUST BEFORE BED

At night, you'll basically be repeating the program, but with a
few differences. For one thing, you won't be shaving. On the
other hand, you may have a genuinely dirty face. If the latter
is true, read step one, below; if not, skip directly to step two.

(1) If your face is very grimy, the result of much perspir-
ing, of a build-up of dirt, or for whatever reason, you can

wash it with a little shaving cream. Take some in the palm of your hand, make a lather and apply it to the face; then rinse thoroughly with lukewarm water. (Shaving cream, provided it's unscented and unmentholated, is not nearly as alkaline—and, hence, as drying—as soap. While you shouldn't use it regularly, it is safe for those occasions when a major cleansing is in order.) If you like, you can follow this with a simple balancing lotion made of one half teaspoon of borax *or* one tablespoon of white vinegar or lemon juice to four cups of tap water. Make sure the water is neither hot nor cold but is at room temperature. If you are a bronzer wearer, or if you are a model or actor who has to wear even heavier forms of makeup, you should begin with a full-fledged cleansing cream. (Again, see the formulary for a good basic one.) This cleans more deeply than the cleansing lotion, and also cuts the grease on which most makeup products are based. Apply to your face and massage gently into the skin. Tissue off. Repeat until the most recent tissue comes up clean.

(2) Apply cleansing lotion, as in the morning.

(3) Rinse your face and neck with lukewarm tap water.

(4) Apply eye cream, as in the morning.

(5) Apply before/after shave moisturizer, as in the morning. Or, if your skin is feeling slightly dry—on account of cold weather, for instance—use a night cream (see formulary), which is a much richer and more nourishing substance. Massage the cream gently but firmly into the skin, avoiding the nose and chin area unless they, too, are excessively dry. Blot off excess with a tissue.

Men with skin that is both dry and dehydrated should—at least in the coldest weather—apply the night cream, then *follow* with a coating of before/after shave moisturizer, over the entire surface of the face and neck, so that it completely covers the night cream, as well as the nose and chin. Finish with a spray of bottled spring water, and pat dry. Of course, if you're pressed for time, you needn't undertake this procedure every single night; you can use either the night cream *or* the moisturizer and still be adequately protected.

Men with oily skin in general should not use their before/after shave moisturizer at bedtime, but they can apply a little to those spots where their face feels particularly dry or irritated. I don't believe that anyone with oily skin should ever use a night cream. Oily skin simply doesn't need that much lubrication. It needs, instead, to breathe.

SPECIAL TREATS AND TREATMENTS
Facial

You'll remember that I promised a more rigorous program at bedtime because the skin renews itself during sleep. Well, *every* bedtime needn't be rigorous, provided you follow the steps of your skin-care regimen faithfully. Still, you may want to do something special, something more far-reaching for your face at this relatively relaxed time of the day. In Chapter VIII I'll describe a full facial massage, designed to stimulate the oil glands of dry and normal skins and to help regulate their activity, providing the skin with both the lubrication it needs if it's to be supple and the moisture it habitually requires. (Oily skins have their own facial, and *that* one I'll get to in just a minute.) This facial should be undertaken only after the face has been thoroughly cleansed, and it should be followed with the customary applications of eye cream and night cream (with or without moisturizer).

The facial is the most far-reaching technique at your disposal. But precisely because it's so far-reaching, it's also time-consuming: the full facial can easily take half an hour.

For those nights when there's enough time to do something more than just the usual cleansing and lubricating, yet not enough time to go the whole facial massage route, consider a mask. All facials conclude with this process, anyway, and it is extraordinarily refreshing, cleansing, and invigorating for your spirits as well as your skin. Moreover, it shouldn't take more than ten minutes.

The After-Shave Mask

The most basic mask you can give yourself I choose to call the after-shave mask, and there is no question but that it is most effective when applied to the face after shaving, in the morning. However, if you don't have the time or inclination in those early morning hours, it can still do considerable good when applied before you go to bed, counteracting severe irritations such as rashes and pimples. Just as important, it can help tone the skin of the entire face and neck area, deep-cleansing it, as well as stimulating blood circulation as the mask tightens in the course of setting. Most noticeably, it will give your skin a healthy glow and leave your face feeling refreshed.

You can make your own after-shave mask by combining a base of powdered clay (in my New York salon, I call this substance at-home powder) with your own specially formulated liquid to make a paste, which you'll then apply directly to your face. You'll find the formula for at-home powder in the formulary. To one level tablespoon of the powder in a bowl, simply add enough of your cleansing lotion or before/after shave moisturizer to make a creamy paste, neither so thick as to seem heavy nor so thin as to be runny. Apply all over your face and neck, and let set for anywhere from five to twenty minutes—the longer you leave it on, the more pronounced its effect will be. Avoid the eye area, which is too delicate to be subjected to the mask's drying tendencies. And make sure, if your neck is dry, that you pre-treat it with eye or night cream.

Since the mask tightens as it dries, it's always a good idea to relax, even lie down, while you have it on. If you talk, eat, or even laugh, if you do *anything* that requires the use of your facial muscles, you'll interfere with the action of the mask. Besides, you risk stretching your skin excessively. After the mask has hardened, rinse it off thoroughly with plenty of cool or lukewarm water (never hot!), then apply before/after shave moisturizer (or night cream, if your skin is not oily and you prefer the extra richness it affords). Let me stress again that while this mask is specially formulated to be used after shaving, it will serve your complexion equally well at any time of the day or night. Use it when you feel that there's enough time for you to treat yourself to something, or whenever you really want to look your best.

That's the simplest mask at your disposal. However, I suggest that you turn to the formulary and read over the formulas for a couple of others in the section devoted to your skin type. Masks come in many different variations, and while most of the ones I recommend are based on this at-home formula, you can vary the other ingredients to play up certain of the mask's inherent capabilities. You can emphasize the toning effect, for instance, or the nourishing one, or the hydrating one. Which one you choose will depend on the state of your skin at any given moment, as well as on the ingredients you happen to have handy.

Wheat Bran or Cornmeal Peels

Another shortcut routine is the superficial wheat bran or cornmeal peel. (Dry and normal complexions use the former, oily ones the latter.) This streamlined cleansing treatment can do much to improve your looks. Its deep-cleansing action removes part of the superficial layer of dead cells on the surface of the skin. Since these dead cells tend to asphyxiate the skin, even their partial removal results in a better oxygen supply to the deeper cell layers. The skin's metabolism is improved, and since the newly exposed cells are better hydrated, you'll see an immediate improvement in the look of your skin as well. Stimulation from the peeling massage improves blood and lymph flow, too, so the face looks less congested, and any oily accretions, such as blackheads, resulting from clogged pores, are unblocked.

Check the formulary to find out how to make your own wheat bran or cornmeal peel. The steps for using it are very simple. First cleanse your skin well with cleansing lotion, rinsing afterwards with lukewarm water. Then apply the paste all over the face and neck, except around the eyes. Massage for two minutes by pinching the cheek and jaw areas gently between your thumb and second or third finger. It is important to keep your touch light, so as not to damage the skin in any way. (And never administer a superficial peel to skin troubled by pimples or infections.)

Then, with light, rapid, circular movements, massage the entire face and neck with the third fingers of both hands, starting at the neck and working up to the forehead (again avoiding the eye and under-eye areas). Pay special attention to the sides of the nose.

Let the paste set: on an oily face for between five and ten minutes; on a dry or normal one for only a couple of minutes, *not* more. Then rinse it off, and apply, if you wish, the aftershave mask for your skin type for between ten and twenty minutes. This will prove especially beneficial if your skin is reddish, splotchy, or otherwise irritated. Rinse the mask off (always use cool or lukewarm water) and apply your before/after shave moisturizer. Your skin will look clean, refreshed, and revitalized. Small wrinkles will be less visible, and the flakiness that so often plagues a dry skin or the sallowness typical of an oily one will disappear. Caution, though: this process is so rigorous that it shouldn't be undertaken by anybody—especially if his skin is sensitive—more than once a week.

The Facial for Oily Skin

I want to take a minute or two to counsel the man with very oily skin, whose needs are greater than those of other men. If your skin *is* chronically, problematically oily, I suggest you skip the at-home facial outlined in Chapter VIII, and substitute this special treatment, which I will give to you in clear, step-by-step fashion. Admittedly, the special treatment takes a bit of time, but it's well worth the effort; it will help your skin slough accumulated dead cells, will cleanse and tighten pores, and relieve sallowness and skin congestion. You need give yourself the special treatment only once a week; in between you can maintain the improvements wrought by your new regimen with the simple application of a mask, as described above.

Please note again that the special treatment for oily skin is intended only for men with very oily skin who are not plagued by acne. (If you do have acne, you'll want to read about at-home remedial measures in the chapter on acne.) Now let's begin.

(1) Cleanse your face thoroughly with cotton balls dipped in cleansing lotion, using several applications, until no dirt shows up on the cotton.

(2) Combine cornmeal available in health food stores and supermarkets with enough water to make a paste, and apply the paste over the entire face, avoiding, however, the eye area. Use your fingertips to massage in a light, circular motion. Then rinse off the paste with plenty of lukewarm water. This paste acts as a scrub to remove dead cells from your skin's surface. (This, of course, is the by now familiar superficial peel.)

(3) Steam your face for about ten minutes, using a simple steam bath made by steeping a small amount of chamomile tea (available in health food stores) in two cups of boiling water. Use a large saucepan, remove it from the flame and put it on a secure, flat surface. Hold your face about six inches above the saucepan, covering both your head and the pan with a large towel so that the steam can't escape. This steaming process will open your pores and flush oily accretions out of the skin.

(4) Make compresses using a special formula—the supercleansing lotion for oily skin—and large pieces of cotton. The supercleansing lotion is easily made by mixing one teaspoon of baking soda with five ounces (or ten tablespoons) of water. Dip the cotton in the lotion, apply to face, and lie down with the compresses on your face for about ten minutes. (The only reason why you should lie down is to keep the compresses from falling off.) The purpose of this step is to soften any dirt and sebum that are clogging the pores, making them easier to remove.

(5) Once you've taken off the compresses, you can proceed to remove dirt and oil deposits from the pores, using a simple massage technique. Grasp small sections of the skin between the thumb and the knuckles of the forefinger and begin making gentle (I repeat, gentle!) half-rotation movements. Do this over the entire face, again avoiding the eye area, and alternating with a light pinching movement. Keep this up for between five and ten minutes.

(6) Repeat step number one, making sure you cleanse thoroughly.

(7) Apply the after-shave mask, which you'll find, of course, in the formulary at the back of the book, using any of the appropriate additions. Leave it on for fifteen minutes,

then rinse off with lukewarm water. Do not apply the mask to the area around the eyes.

The best time to give yourself the special treatment is at night before you go to bed. Your skin, like your body, renews itself while you sleep, and this will allow it several hours to rest, breathe, and reap the full benefits of the treatment. If this is impossible, you can, of course, give yourself the special treatment whenever it is most convenient.

As I said before, you need to use the special treatment only once a week. In between, say two or three times a week, you can skip right to the final step, the mask, which will give your skin many of the same cleansing and refreshing benefits in much less time.

Dehydrated Oily Skin

Many men with oily skin nevertheless have dehydrated skin, as well. As you might imagine, a dehydrated oily skin has all the typical signs of an ordinary oily skin, i.e., the thickness and the visible pores. But there is, in addition, a network of lines, or superficial wrinkles, very thin and small in appearance, that traces all over the face, especially around areas of facial expression, the neck, the sides of the cheek near the ears, and in the area just below and behind the ear lobe. Dehydration can nullify the advantages of having oily skin altogether, since it will age you as much and as rapidly as having dry skin would.

Luckily, however, dehydration is much easier to eliminate in your case, since nine times out of ten it is caused only by using soap or other harsh cleansers, too-strong astringents commonly recommended for oily skin, and highly alcoholic after-shaves or colognes. Changing your cleansing routine, especially your shaving routine, and with it your products, can improve dehydration overnight. (If you had a dry skin, the problem would be more difficult to solve, since dry skin lacks a moisture-retaining oil barrier.) If you think your oily skin is dehydrated, I advise you to begin using the products and routines already outlined, and follow the suggestions for shaving in Chapter VII, remembering always to apply before/after shave emulsion to any dehydrated areas of the face.

Another possibility is to use a particularly emollient cleansing lotion. You might add collagen, double the fructose or honey content, and add a full two or three tablespoons of Aloe Vera gel to the recommended oily-skin cleansing lotion formula in the formulary. (Aloe Vera gel and hydrolized collagen are available at most health food stores.) Used overnight, this upgraded formula will give you more than adequate protection.

If, after a month or so of using these products, your skin still seems dehydrated, however, the cause may be more complicated. Quick-weight-loss diets, which dehydrate the body, will also wreak havoc on your skin cells, as will diuretics (popularly known as water pills) and many other prescription drugs. Low atmospheric humidity, such as you'll find in any artificially heated or air-conditioned room, will also dry out an otherwise healthy skin. The solutions to these problems are simple: stop taking any drugs that aren't absolutely necessary to your survival, get a room humidifier, at least for your bedroom or your office, and continue to cleanse and hydrate your skin in the ways we've discussed. The problem should begin to clear up immediately.

When Skin Is Both Dry and Dehydrated

Clearly, it's critical that you take care of your skin. By all means, use both before/after shave emulsion *and* night cream before bed, finishing with a spray of spring water, if you like. In addition, give yourself facial treatments as often as possible; the warm wax mask (see formulary), for instance, is especially well suited to the needs of your eye area.

Finally, if your skin is very dry indeed, you can mix a little eye cream with your moisturizer or with your night cream—mix it right in the palm of your hand—for added richness and emollience.

When Skin Is Sensitive or Irritated

Sensitive skin is frequently a result of insufficient oils. Of course, our whole dry-skin regimen is designed to counteract that condition, to get the oil glands functioning as normally as possible. But if your own sensitivity is great enough, you can, in the meantime, assuage it with an oil compress every three or four days.

Make a mask, with holes for the eyes, nose, and mouth, out of a soft white cloth—cotton, say, or flannel. It should be roughly the shape of your face and neck, so that oil won't get in your hair (where it will prove hard to wash out). Preheat some olive, peanut, or corn oil, dip the mask in the oil, and apply it to your face for twenty minutes, while you lie down and relax. When you remove the mask, lightly massage your face with your fingertips until the oil has completely penetrated the skin. This is as effective for itching, dry, irritated skin as any remedy I know of. But be careful. If your skin is truly sensitive, you may be allergic to one or more of the recommended oils. Always test a new oil on a tiny patch of skin before plunging ahead with it. If you're one of the rare people who is allergic to olive, peanut, and corn oil, you may substitute mineral oil, which won't nourish the skin as the other oils do, but will at least lubricate it.

ONE LAST NOTE

This is your regimen. You own *it*—it doesn't own *you*. Just because your regimen states that you should cleanse your skin twice a day, don't think, for instance, that you can't also cleanse your face at six o'clock in the evening, if you feel it's dirty or even if you just want to refresh yourself. Just make sure that you apply the basic *principles* of the regimen: for instance, if your skin is dry, after cleansing with the lotion, reapply eye cream and before/after shave emulsion; in short, that you lubricate those areas that you've just stripped oil and moisture from in the cleansing process. Likewise, don't hesitate to experiment with the full range of masks for your skin type, finding the ingredient that serves—or perhaps merely pleases—you best. There *is* flexibility here. There has to be. You are a modern man, pressed for time, under pressure, working against all manner of deadlines—physical, professional, psychological. Your regimen, properly handled, won't intensify the pressure. It will help you counter the signs of it. And, in time, it may even reduce the pressure itself.

FOUR

BLACK SKIN

MELANIN, PIGMENT, AND THE SUN

WHAT WE PERCEIVE as skin color—whether it's the result of centuries of racial heritage or of a weekend of sitting in the sun—is, without exception, a function of a protein called melanin, produced in everybody's skin by microscopic structures called melanocytes, situated in the basal layer of the epidermis. Melanin (from the Greek word for black) in a fairly complicated process migrates from this basal layer to the outermost layer of the skin, darkening as it goes, and finally settling down in the form of what we call pigment in the case of the black race, tan in the case of a season at the beach.

Melanin is a wonderful substance. Not only does it cause the striking variations in skin color between races (as well as within them), but also singlehandedly offers protection from the damaging—and potentially deadly—ultraviolet rays of the sun. Blacks, who historically had their origins in the equatorial region of Africa, where the sun is as strong and relentless as it ever gets, naturally had need of greater protection. And they got it. While they have no more melanocytes than the Swedes do, the melanocytes that they do have are more active, producing greater amounts of melanin, rushing it to the surface of the skin, and dispersing it in ways different from its dispersion in white skin. The result of all this zeal on the part of the melanocytes—a zeal that is genetically programmed, I might add, not environmentally triggered—is a rich pigmentation that can range from ebony to tan, and embracing all the gradations in between.

DIFFERENCES BETWEEN BLACK AND WHITE SKIN

Black skin confers a number of advantages, dermatologically speaking. First and foremost, it provides natural resistance to the sun, all of whose deleterious effects you'll read about in the chapter on tanning (Chapter X). In fact, a successful summer tan is simply the effort of white skin to reach the same level of protectiveness that black skin enjoys naturally. Of course, black people *can* get sunburned—and it's as painful for them as for freckle-faced redheads when they do—but much larger doses of sun are required for this to happen.

Because of this natural protection against ultraviolet radiation, black skin is also more resistant to wrinkling and to the disintegration of its collagen, as the sun takes its toll summer after summer. Finally, black skin is more resistant to all forms of skin cancer.

Besides pigment, black skin differs from white skin in two important ways. First, it has, per square inch, more sweat glands; these glands are bigger than those in white skin, too, which means that the pores they terminate in are larger and more noticeable. And the secretion itself—the sweat—is more abundant and even evaporates faster. This means that blacks are better provided for not only against the ultraviolet rays of the sun, which are perceived as light and which cause burning, but against the infrared ones, too, which take the form of heat. The black skin is, in every way, better accommodated to the rigors of a tropical existence, or of a summertime one.

Second, black skin also has larger and more numerous oil glands. Moreover, fully one-tenth of them open directly onto the surface of the skin, whereas in white skin virtually all are situated in the uppermost part of the dermis. This means, again, that pores are larger and more noticeable in black skin than in white, and the oil itself is more abundant. Thus, black skin tends to be well lubricated, and, as a result, to age slower than the majority of the white skin.

SPECIAL PROBLEMS OF BLACK SKIN

On the other hand, black skin is every bit as susceptible to dehydration as white skin. Typically, this manifests itself, among a fairly high percentage of my black clients, in a kind of grayish, even ashy, cast to the complexion. It is, fortunately, a fairly easy problem to solve, whether it occurs on the face itself or virtually anywhere on the upper body. Simply treat as you would any dehydrated skin, using your after-shave emulsion and night cream to lock in the moisture that your skin is so clearly calling out for. I can almost promise you that your skin will regain its healthy color without your ever having to learn the formal name of your condition—pityriasis alba.

Keloids

A much bigger problem among blacks, and especially black men, is keloidal scarring. Keloids are masses of tough, thick, and unsightly scar tissue that can grow over minor skin injuries—pimples, shaving nicks, cosmetic surgery incisions, ingrown hairs (more on this later), almost anything. White people can get keloids too, but no more than 1 percent do; unfortunately, the incidence is much, much higher among blacks. Even more unfortunate is the fact that there's not a lot you can do about this scarring if you are a man who's prone to keloids.

Obviously, keloids can't be removed surgically: that would only lead to more keloids. Sometimes, however, they can be substantially diminished by the injection of steroids directly into the scar by a dermatologist. The most important advice I can give you, though, is to know your own tendency toward keloid reactions. If you do get keloids, by all means avoid all forms of cosmetic surgery, from face-lifts to silicone implantation to dermabrasion. (The latter, especially, which involves—quite literally—the grinding down of the skin, generally to remove acne scars, can transform the face into one giant keloid.) And be on the lookout for any signs of acne; if you think you're developing any, apply the techniques of acne therapy I outline in Chapter V. The best way to handle keloids is obviously to avoid them in the first place, and that's a simple matter of prevention coupled with skin-care discipline.

There is also some evidence that adequate doses of Vitamin E can prevent and/or help heal keloids. The late Adelle Davis, in her book *Let's Get Well*, states that at least 200 IU of Vitamin E taken internally every day, coupled with topical applications of it direct from the capsule to affected areas of the skin, will, in most cases, bring about noticeable, scar-free clearing. She speculates that blacks may have an especially high nutritional requirement for Vitamin E. (If you don't like vitamin capsules, by the way, you can increase your Vitamin E intake by eating plenty of lettuce, avocados, corn oil, and wheat germ.)

Ingrown Hairs

Before I leave the subject of keloids altogether, let me address myself to the issue of shaving, a special problem for some black men, and a prime factor in keloid formation, for, among those so afflicted, every little nick and every ingrown hair can result in the formation of new scar tissue. Ingrown hairs are generally a problem only in those areas that you shave. When a hair is cut flush with the skin surface, its microscopic spiraling can cause it to grow back into the skin. The coarser and curlier the hairs, the more likely they are to become ingrown; this means, obviously, that ingrown hairs are a much more common complaint among black men than white, although the latter can also be susceptible. Ingrown hairs can result not only in keloids, but in shaving bumps, rashes, and inflammations of various kinds.

What can you do about ingrown hairs? I recommend that you observe the following shaving precautions. First, shave not against, but *with* the growth of your beard. Second, rather than closely, shave *frequently;* this means the individual hairs, even when freshly cut, won't lie quite so flush with the skin's surface, which means, in turn, that it will be that much harder for them to find reentry. Third, always make sure that your blade, whether manual or electric, is very sharp. And if your ingrown hairs are accompanied by inflammation, you should see a doctor.

Depilatories and Electrolysis

If you have an ingrown hair problem so severe that no amount of simple shaving technique seems to help, you may have no recourse but to use a chemical depilatory to remove the hairs altogether. In general, depilatories in powder form are more efficient than those in cream form; and you also have the option of mixing such powder, not with water, but with a *very* strong chamomile tea, which will make the whole process considerably less irritating to your complexion. (Simply steep three chamomile tea bags in half of a cup of hot water for at least fifteen minutes before mixing the resulting liquid with the depilatory powder.) The night before you apply the depilatory, always use a moisturizer (even if you have oily skin and aren't a regular moisturizer user). In the morning, apply the depilatory right over that layer of moisturizer. After you rinse off the paste, cleanse thoroughly with cleansing lotion and re-apply the moisturizer. And never use a depilatory more than every other day; such products can irritate even ordinarily cooperative complexions. Alternatives to depilatories are electrolysis and the process called Depilatron. The former consists of inserting an extremely fine needle into the hair follicle itself and feeding an electrical current through it; essentially, the follicle is being electrocuted. Depilatron is a somewhat less radical, and somewhat safer means of getting rid of unwanted hair. No needles are used; in fact nothing enters or even touches the skin. Rather, a trained technician applies special tweezers to the individual hairs *above* the skin, which removes the hair *and* weakens its growth cells back in the follicle. The skin is not damaged, nor is it shocked. Whichever method you choose, you'll of course want to see a specialist. And bear in mind that, while more expensive than depilatories, both electrolysis and Depilatron can be permanent in time.

Pigmentation

Finally, black men face the threat of problems that are pigment-related. Not that they derive from the degree of pigmentation, necessarily; it's just that several skin conditions are more noticeable there. Others, while hardly restricted to blacks, *are* more prevalent among them. Postinflammatory hypopigmentation, for instance, refers to the tendency on the part of black skin to lighten noticeably in color after acute inflammation—the kind that might result from rashes or burns, psoriasis, or simple acne. Unfortunately, there's very little that can be done about it. On the other hand, if you suffer from the opposite of this condition, namely, hyperpigmentation (or, more simply, darkening), you can apply a cream that contains a bleaching agent, like hydroquinone. Always use such a preparation in combination with a good tanning lotion (see chapter X), as exposure to the sun—and the production of extra melanin that it triggers—makes hyperpigmentation worse. And if you suffer from acne, you should realize that the chemical resorcin, which is very common in commercial acne preparations, can darken black skin. Check the label of any medicine you might buy to make sure it doesn't contain resorcin, if hyperpigmentation is a problem for you.

As for taking care of your skin, well, that's pretty much a matter of following the appropriate regimens, as they've been laid out in Chapters I, II, and III. But men with black skin are especially likely to have oily skin as well—the result of the abundance of sebaceous glands I mentioned early in this chapter. In this case, the basic goals of the regimen are the same as for any oily-skin regimen: thorough cleansing and the conscientious removing of all excess surface oil, toning, and the sloughing of dead cells that clog the complexion and make it sallow or ashen. The last goal is especially important, as black skin is a thick skin and tends to shed its dead cells at a quicker rate than white skin. However, much of the black skin I have examined over the years is just as likely to be dry or, on rare occasions, to exist in that wonderful state called normal. Most frequently, it will be, just like white skin, combination—with areas of oiliness *and* areas of dryness and/or normalcy. In each case, it should be treated according to the appropriate regimens already provided in this book.

———•———

FIVE

ACNE

A CNE CAN BE one of the major ordeals of adolescence, as we all know, but it doesn't necessarily disappear with the teens; often it extends into the twenties and beyond and, unless it is properly treated, it can leave scars that last a lifetime. Early recognition and treatment can bring any case under control, however, and avert all possibility of scarring.

WHAT IT IS

When we speak of acne, we usually mean a condition typified by blackheads, whiteheads, pimples, and clogged pores on the face, back, or chest. This is technically referred to as acne juvenalis, or, in adults, acne vulgaris. No one knows exactly what causes acne, but we do have a fairly good idea of how it works. The mainspring is an erratic overactivity of the sebaceous, or oil, glands which lie beneath the surface of the skin. This overactivity is probably caused by the hormonal and glandular changes that accompany the onset of puberty, but any number of factors can cause it later in life. While the sebaceous glands are producing oil, or sebum, at a very fast rate, much of this sebum never reaches the surface of the skin, where it could be routinely washed away. Instead, it becomes trapped in the pores that open onto the surface of the skin. Sebum can become trapped for a number of reasons: there may be so much cellular debris on the surface of the skin that the pore is covered by a physical, though barely visible, barrier; or the pore opening may not be large enough for the accretion of sebum to pass through. More often, however, the problem is the characteristically stiff, waxy, form of the sebum itself. No longer fluid, it becomes thick enough to form a rod up to a quarter inch long. At the surface of the skin this rod or plug can manifest itself in four different ways: as a blackhead, whitehead, pimple, or clogged pore.

Blackheads

A blackhead (or comedo—the plural is comedones) is a plug that just reaches the surface of the skin, but cannot go any farther. There, the oil oxidizes on contact with the air, turning the tip of the plug black. Blackheads are sometimes covered with an opaque layer of cellular debris, but they are still recognizable as blackheads (pimples and whiteheads are raised higher on the surface of the skin). Strong abrasive scrubs, which I do not recommend, or polyester web sponges, which are even worse, can sometimes remove the tip of the blackhead. But because the plug itself, which lodges deep inside the skin, is not removed, it regains its black appearance in a couple of days or so.

Whiteheads

A whitehead is usually the precursor to a pimple. Here the rod or plug of sebum completely misses the pore opening. Still it pushes upward onto the surface of the skin, where it forms a raised bump, more or less white in appearance depending on the pigmentation of the skin, but without the surrounding redness and white point of a pimple. Whiteheads are most difficult to extract without trauma to the skin—they can only be properly removed by a specialist. If it contains pus, a whitehead will soon develop into a pimple, at which point it becomes easier to extract.

Pimples

A pimple usually appears as a red spot with a small white center, or head, in which the pus is formed by a reaction of sebum with irritating enzymes and microbes. Pimples that are left untreated usually become further infected, causing more inflammation, more pus, and usually, enlargement of the affected site. Sometimes a pimple will rupture into the surrounding tissues. This is one of the worst dangers of improper squeezing; the result can be an enlarged, pitted scar that remains even after the lesion finally heals. If you catch them early enough, however, these blemishes need never be permanent. Visit the nearest dermatologist or skin-care clinic at the first sign of them.

Clogged Pores

Clogged or asphyxiated pores look like blackheads minus the black spot; in this case the sebum plug does not oxidize, although there may be adjacent blackheads. There is no head and usually no surrounding redness or irritation, because clogged pores are not infected and no pus has been formed. They can, however, become infected and turn into pimples if they are not removed. And even if they don't turn into pimples, neglect may cause the pore to become permanently enlarged.

ACNE THERAPY

If you have acne, *do* something about it. I think the most harmful fallacy concerning acne is that nothing can lessen or prevent it. Nine out of ten cases can either be cured or brought under control in a matter of months, and even the stubbornest case is not hopeless. I find it tragic that teenagers allow their faces to become disfigured just because they don't know they can be helped, or because they have been misinformed. Acne treatment requires specialized knowledge that only a skin-care specialist or dermatologist can give you; many family doctors simply aren't equipped to deal with it.

Another dangerous notion about acne is that products or drugs alone are enough to clear it up. This is just not true. Until every acne accretion has been manually removed from the skin, there can be no hope of eliminating the condition. Such work can take a long time. In acute cases, ten, twenty, or more one-hour sessions are necessary. Many dermatologists are unwilling to do this tedious work themselves. The good ones, however, will have either a skin-care technician or nurse trained in skin care in their office to do it, or they will recommend a good skin-care clinic or salon where the work can be done.

Sometimes a dermatologist will tell you that acne does not have to be treated manually; that drugs, antibiotics, abrasive or caustic products, surgery, chemical peelings, or just time will take care of the problem. In this case, your best bet is to find another dermatologist. Likewise, if your family physician (who may be an excellent doctor in other respects) gives you a prescription for tetracycline or some other oral antibiotic, telling you just to take the pills and not touch your face, seek more specialized advice. These antibiotics can have profound side effects and they should never be administered to an acne patient until every less potentially dangerous avenue of treatment has been explored. Remember, every case of acne is different, and those who respond to one treatment may not respond to another. I myself have never seen a case in which antibiotics could not be avoided. Moreover, most acne sufferers will need some kind of supportive treatments for quite a while after the problem has been controlled. Relying on antibiotics for such long-term support can have serious consequences for your health.

Effective acne therapy consists of two essential parts: use of the correct products, and proper manual treatment.

Products

The acne-type skin should be cleansed two or three times daily. I prefer a slightly acidic astringent lotion with an alcoholic content between 40 and 50 percent, but no more. A higher alcoholic content (say 80 percent), or stronger solvents, such as benzene, acetone (nail polish remover, which is actually found in some acne lotions), or carbon tetrachloride, should never be used because of their strong dehydrating effect and their excessive degreasing action. Dehydration will cause premature wrinkling and sagging of the face; this is why people using such products seem to have such dry, flaky skin, when in fact their skin is physiologically oily. When these products have cracked and dried the skin, more oil is trapped beneath the skin surface resulting in further eruptions that are even harder to remove. Dehydration also causes crevices in which dirt particles can lodge, and heightens irritation, which can also cause more pimples.

If the skin is completely degreased, the sebaceous glands will tend to react by producing more oil than ever. Producing oil is their job, and when you take every trace of oil off the skin, you are giving the glands the signal to go into action.

Because surface irritation can overstimulate the sebaceous glands, soothing ingredients are an important part of the cleansing lotion. If you use soap—even an acne soap—to cleanse the face, an acid-balanced lotion must be used afterwards to restore acidity and remove traces of waxy emulsifier that will further irritate the skin.

Finally, since staphylococcal infection may be present in the pustules, the lotion must be antiseptic; moreover, because it is acid, the lotion assists the skin's own bacteria-fighting acid system. As you will see, I recommend ingredients such as witch hazel, camphor, sulphur, boric acid, and alum in the acne lotion formula in the formulary.

Other products necessary to support acne therapy include disinfectant powders that can be used after shaving and ointments containing vitamins to promote scarless healing of the skin. In addition, bacteriostatic ointments or creams such as Bacitracin may be used. Under the guidance of your dermatologist, you may also use ointments containing other agents such as hydrocortisone, or antiyeast and antifungal (as well as bacteriostatic) agents such as Mycolog cream, which are only available on prescription. Of late, Vitamin A acid (retinoic acid) has become a popular treatment with many dermatologists, though it, like other acne remedies, tends to dry the outer layers of the skin excessively. Of course, every new agent that becomes available offers the acne specialist more scope in finding a treatment that will work effectively for you. My feeling, however, is that given a chance, the older, more conservative remedies usually work best and pose far less danger of systemic toxicity than newer drugs that have not yet been thoroughly studied. Whoever is treating your skin should be familiar with all therapeutic agents, old and new. Too often, the attitude is that "new is best" and of course, it is always more exciting for the practitioner to use a new product on his patients. But there is no miracle product for acne. Patient use of conservative products plus manual treatment invariably brings the best results.

Manual Treatment

It may seem a bit severe to say that manual treatment of the skin by a skin-care specialist or dermatologist is mandatory for all acne sufferers, but I believe there are no exceptions to this rule. I have seen so many teen-agers with infections brought on by careless squeezing that I cannot, with honesty, tell you anything else. These conditions are especially tragic when the case is so far advanced that scars are inevitable, when treatment even a few months earlier could have prevented them. One young man came to me only when his face was so covered with pimples that it was impossible for him to shave any part of his face or neck without cutting one. Needless to say, many months of treatment were necessary before his condition cleared up. Why did he, like many others, wait so long before seeking help? Few people realize that regular treatment following the very first signs of blackheads and pimples can reduce acne to the status of a minor annoyance rather than a serious medical problem. Regular acne treatment cuts blemish production to an absolute minimum and promotes rapid healing of the few blemishes that are unavoidable. Depending on the case, treatment may be necessary once a week, or only once every two months. It may be hard for you to find a good acne specialist in your area, or you may consider the treatments too expensive. But every acne sufferer should make the effort to have his condition treated properly; the rewards of a blemish-free complexion are great, and so are the risks of neglect.

All impurities of the skin must be cleaned out regularly. A dermatologist or skin-care specialist does this by squeezing, preferably after careful pretreatment. Why shouldn't you do the squeezing yourself? Because there is a specific technique for squeezing, and this technique requires an expertise that comes only with long years of practice. Improper squeezing is dangerous. For one thing, if you are too rough (and almost everyone is), you will injure the tissue surrounding the pustule, causing capillaries to break. By using incorrect movements, you can also cause adjacent pimples to rupture into the deeper skin layers, spreading the infection. The most serious objection to at-home squeezing, however, is that few nonspecialists can gauge exactly when every trace of pus and sebum has been eliminated from the pore. In many cases, getting everything out requires considerable manual skill.

Some amateur squeezers do get everything out but, not knowing they have, they continue to squeeze, causing severe damage to the tissues. Most of the time, though, some trace of pus or sebum is left in the pore. This causes another, and usually more severe, blemish to form in the same spot. One reason why professional treatment is so successful compared to at-home tinkering is precisely the fact that blemishes are completely removed and cannot reappear again and again in the same place.

Before-and-After Treatment

One important and frequently overlooked aspect of squeezing is the before-and-after treatment. Good dermatologists and skin-care clinics will always provide this invaluable service. Briefly, pretreatment is a procedure taking approximately twenty minutes, the purpose of which is to make the skin more receptive to squeezing. First, the skin is deep-cleansed with preparations that emulsify fatty accretions deep in the skin layers and dissolve the dead cells which make blemishes more difficult to remove. Then the face is steamed for ten minutes to relax the pores, further loosen the blemishes, and bring impurities to the surface of the skin. Often, special disincrustation products are also used to soften the outer crust that is so typical of maltreated acne skin. By making blemishes significantly easier to extract, this procedure minimizes the risk of mechanical injury or trauma.

Postextraction treatment is most essential. Once blemishes have been removed, the face must be thoroughly disinfected to prevent new infection or the spread of an existing one. Then an astringent mask, usually based on clay, is applied. This further disinfects, closes the pores, promotes healing, soothes the skin, and restores the protective acid mantle. Creams and lotions to disinfect the skin and promote healing can be based on agents such as zinc oxide, sulphur, camphor, calamine, kaoline, or bentonite. Mild antiirritant agents, contained in camphor and chamomile extracts, are especially important to counteract shaving irritation. You can buy camphor in block or powder form or as spirits of camphor at your drugstore. Chamomile is available in health food stores.

FIRST AID

I realize there will be times when you will need a pimple to be squeezed, especially when the pus has broken out through the head, and you will not, for whatever reason, be able to see a dermatologist or skin-care specialist. I can try to teach you how to squeeze properly, but I must warn you that there is always the risk of manual trauma and infection, although these can be minimized by the correct procedures and products. But first, to daily cleansing.

Cleansing

I would advise you not to use soap because of its alkaline qualities and the necessity of using an acid rinse afterwards. A special acne cleansing lotion (see Formulary) will do a good job of thoroughly cleansing and soothing an acne-type skin without excessive degreasing or dehydration.

The lotion is applied with pieces of cotton torn from a roll, or with cotton balls. Use two or three pieces of cotton, until you can see no trace of dirt on them. Cleanse in the morning only, after shaving (see Chapter VII). Instead of using before/after shave moisturizer, use the special antiirritant shaving cream, also discussed in Chapter VII, for your five minute pretreatment prior to shaving, if you are using the wet blade method. After shaving and rinsing off the cream, apply the lotion. If you are using an electric shaver (the best of these can be very valuable for acned skin), you won't need to use the lotion first unless your face is too oily for a comfortable shave, but always use the lotion afterwards.

Cleanse at night before going to bed, and during the day only if the face is excessively greasy.

Using an antiseptic powder every day after shaving can be very helpful when applied to affected areas of the face—to the beard area if irritated, and to all acne sites. You will find two such powders in the formulary in the back of the book.

Using the after-shave mask for acne (see Formulary) every day can be a great boon in your treatment. The more consistently you use it, the faster you'll get relief, but don't use it more than once a day. It should be applied immediately after shaving, and left on the skin for fifteen to twenty minutes. Rinse it off with cool, not cold water, pat the face dry with a tissue, and apply cleansing lotion. Remember never to apply cleansing lotion or masks to the eye area. If you cannot use the mask in the morning, use it when you come home at night. It can also be dotted over pimples before you go to bed, and rinsed off with cleansing lotion in the morning.

Ointments

At night you can apply a zinc oxide ointment, two variations of which appear in the formulary.

These ointments, with their content of Vitamins A, D, and E, disinfect the skin, help to eliminate scarring, and promote healing. Topical applications of Vitamin E can also be extremely helpful. Vitamin E works best when incorporated as an ingredient in a moisturizer or a cream; pure Vitamin E oil is very sticky and doesn't penetrate the skin easily. In my experience, Vitamin E smooths the skin, calms irritations, and can have a healing effect even on existing scar tissue. I myself have had consistently good results with it and, contrary to the claims of some of its detractors, I have never seen it produce an allergic reaction.

ACNE   77

To get back to our zinc oxide ointment, it should be applied only to affected areas of the skin, i.e. where there is redness, irritation, or a blemish. Ointment #2 is stronger and should be used less frequently. Both versions are stable, so you can make small batches and use them on alternate nights or alternate weeks. This brings us to an important fact in treating acne: frequently acne will respond to a product very well, but only for a short time, perhaps a month or so. By alternating products, you don't give the skin a chance to become accustomed to a particular active agent, so the chances of its not working are lessened. If you are seeing a dermatologist, you might alternate these ointments with a stronger prescription he recommends. This will minimize the risks of these stronger products, namely destruction of the beneficial skin flora that help to fight infection, and toxicities that are often discovered only after a product has been on the market for years. Generally speaking, it is safer to use products based on vitamins and natural minerals, such as zinc and sulphur.

Whatever external ointment you apply to your face, remember to use it only on areas that are affected by acne.

Squeezing Pimples, Blackheads, and Clogged Pores

Now to the proper way to squeeze pimples. This is a variant of the extra cleaning treatments in Chapter VIII, none of which is appropriate for acne. It includes important pre- and post-squeezing steps, and will take between thirty and forty-five minutes. This may strike you as rather time-consuming, but it is the only way to ensure safety and ease of extraction. Please don't take any shortcuts.

(1) Cleanse face and neck thoroughly with calamine lotion, using several pieces of cotton to do so. Rinse well and pat face dry with a clean tissue.

(2) Apply disincrustation compress. This is an alkaline compress made by combining one level teaspoon of baking

soda (sodium bicarbonate) with five ounces (ten table-spoons) of water. Now take strips of cotton torn from a one-pound roll and soak these thoroughly in the solution. Apply to all areas of the face for ten to fifteen minutes. (It is best to lie down while the compress is on, simply to keep it from fall-ing off.)

(3) Remove the compress. Bring a large pot of water to the boil (you can throw in a few spoonfuls or teabags of chamomile flowers, which contain an oil with marked sooth-ing properties, capable of being vaporized and of penetrating the skin). Remove the pot from the flame, and hold your face about twelve inches above it. Drape a large bath towel over your head so that it covers the pot, allowing no steam to es-cape. Adjust your position so that the steam is very warm but not uncomfortably hot. Remain over the pot for five to fifteen minutes, the longer the better.

(4) Now sit or stand in front of a good mirror with a strong light on your face. Pat the face dry with a tissue. Then wrap the second fingers of both hands with small pieces of tissue. Start with the pimples. Only those with well-defined heads are ready to squeeze. Whiteheads, or pimples on which heads have not yet formed, should never be squeezed.

Place the tips of the second fingers right next to the pim-ple. First press *downwards* around the pimple with firm but gentle movements, then press across and into the pimple. Never use excessive force. Squeeze until the sebum and pus have been removed from the follicle, but don't oversqueeze. If a small amount of blood runs out of the follicle, don't squeeze any further (unless there is clearly more pus in the follicle), but go on to the next pimple.

Next, squeeze any large blackheads in exactly the same manner. Blackheads don't usually bleed, but be sure to get all the sebum out, or another blackhead may appear in the same place, and the pore will remain enlarged instead of closing properly.

Finally, squeeze any large, well-defined clogged pores. If the pore seems to be enlarged, has a white plug in the center, but looks neither like a blackhead nor a pimple, it is clogged. Again, all the sebum must be removed, without force.

A note about needles: Some dermatologists recommend using a well-sterilized needle for poking a hole in the roof of pimples or blackheads. If this is done, the needle must never be inserted downward, into the skin, but across the raised surface of the blemish. This can be of some assistance before you squeeze a pimple or blackhead, since it makes a hole through which the pus and sebum can escape. It is most helpful when there is so much cellular debris covering the surface of the affected pore that excessive force would have to be used to squeeze the blemish out. I would incline never to use a needle at home, and to only squeeze pimples and blackheads that will come out of their pores with relative ease, leaving the more stubborn ones to your skin-care specialist. You always run the risk of puncturing the skin. However, if you are careful to follow the recommended procedure, never puncturing the side of the pimple or blackhead more than once, you will be reasonably safe. The needle is only used for blemishes that are raised above the surface of the skin. As I have noted, it must *never* be inserted downward, into the skin, and it must always be disinfected with alcohol first.

Never squeeze for more than fifteen minutes at a time. If there are more clogged pores and blackheads to be taken care of, wait at least three days before giving yourself another treatment. All pimples with definite heads that appear at a given time must be removed, however, so if this takes more than fifteen minutes (it will usually take less than five) continue until they are all removed.

(5) When the squeezing is finished, thoroughly disinfect the face with three or four applications of cleansing lotion.

(6) Apply disinfectant powder number two to all areas of the face except the eyes. Gently dab it on with a small piece of cotton.

(7) Finally, apply the at-home mask for acne, again to the face and neck, not the eye area, and let it dry for ten to twenty minutes. Apply it in a thick layer, using the full quantity.

(8) Rinse off mask with tepid water and blot dry with a tissue. Again apply disinfectant cleansing lotion, and blot dry.

(9) Dot each spot you squeezed with calamine lotion, applied with a Q-tip.

(10) After you clean your face at night, apply zinc oxide ointment—preferably number two—to the spots you have squeezed.

(11) When you clean your face in the morning, apply antiseptic powder to the spots that have been squeezed.

I would advise you to follow this treatment routine only when it is absolutely impossible for you to have your face treated professionally. Results simply cannot be guaranteed otherwise.

This caution administered, however, I think you will find the results of this treatment satisfactory, especially when compared to what happens when you just squeeze your face with dirty hands, without proper disinfection, and without the important before and after treatment. You can avoid nearly all possibility of infection by regular use of the zinc oxide ointment and the antiseptic powder, and if you are careful, you won't have trouble with scarring, especially if your nutrition is adequate.

Regular treatment of acne skin gradully removes infection and impurities. This may take time—perhaps several months—but with the right care, treatments as often as needed, and daily use of the correct products, it is possible to bring all cases of acne vulgaris or juvenalis under control. By this I mean that although the glandular secretions will still be strong, you will only be troubled by an occasional blemish, since deep cleansing prevents blackheads and clogged pores from developing into pimples. Use the products mentioned in this chapter whenever you are in doubt as to what is safe. Of course, if your skin-care specialist wishes to alter any aspect of the routine, you should follow his advice, unless you discover, after a generous trial period, that it isn't working.

NUTRITION AND ACNE

Nutrition is vastly important when it comes to acne. It may even be decisive in clearing it up. Since so many cases are ameliorated or cured when nutrition is improved, I have come to the conclusion that many of them were caused by inadequate nutrition in the first place. All nutrients have either a direct or indirect influence on glandular and hormonal health, and all of them must be supplied in the correct amounts.

I can make suggestions for an anti-acne diet based on a cross section of modern nutritionist research. It is up to you, of course, to decide whether or not you have the discipline to turn these suggestions into dietary rules. Only you can get results. Avoid saturated fats—french fries, potato chips, vegetable shortening, butter, cream, and most margarines are out—and eat a minimum of beef, pork, and lamb. You can rely instead on poultry, dairy products, and eggs for protein.

Even better would be to rely entirely on vegetable proteins, but before trying that you should read Francis Moore Lappé's *Diet for a Small Planet* to learn the right way to obtain protein from vegetable sources.

Sugar (see Chapter XI) is our number one nonfood, and should be avoided completely, not least because it is so easily converted into saturated fat. In the wake of modern research, it would be easy to write two or three volumes on the destructive effects of sugar. It has been called "the world's most dangerous food additive." A totally sugarless diet, one containing no refined carbohydrates and rich in vitamin supplements, often spontaneously clears up acne conditions. Some doctors recommend a glucose tolerance test for acne patients. Sugar interferes with calcium absorption and synthesis of B-vitamins by the intestinal bacteria, and increases the need for Vitamin B_6, one of the most important anti-acne vitamins. A lot of evidence is in, and much of it can be found in the sources suggested in the bibliography at the end of the nutrition chapter. You can read this material and come to your own conclusions, so I think that's enough said. Except for one thing: eliminating sugar from your diet isn't simple; it requires a drastic change of habits. It is not merely a matter of cutting out refined sugar—raw sugar and molasses are just as bad. Although fructose and honey are probably less toxic, these too should be avoided in an anti-acne diet. Cookies, cakes, candies, sodas, all desserts, canned and frozen fruit, ketchup and tomato sauces, and a host of processed foods all contain sugar. If you are extremely active and require large amounts of carbohydrates for fuel, more than adequate energy can be obtained from eating whole grains, especially brown rice, millet (of all grains one of the richest in vitamins and minerals), whole wheat bread, and wheat germ. Additional carbohydrates can be otained from fresh vegetables and fruit; however, an acne diet should never contain too much fruit—emphasize grains first. Be sure, though, that you are getting enough Vitamin C, preferably from vegetables, which are less acidic to the body than fruits.

An anti-acne diet should be light; avoid spicy foods, which can overstimulate the oil glands. Foods rich in fiber are important for their ability to improve intestinal function. Many acne conditions can be traced to constipation or even a mildly below-par intestinal condition. Bran and other fibrous foods will not only relieve constipation, they will also help your stomach synthesize B-vitamins. So will a daily intake of yogurt. One of the best breakfast foods is muesli, the Swiss oat-based cereal, mixed with yogurt and perhaps some fresh fruits. It is available in supermarkets and health food stores under the brand name of Familia, but always buy the kind (there are several varieties) that contains no sugar. If you must have additional sweetening, honey can be added to taste. You can also make your own muesli by combining fresh rolled oats (available at health food stores), yogurt, nuts and/or seeds, and fresh fruit. You will find other suggestions for diet in the nutrition chapter.

Cases of acne are often caused or exacerbated by iodine, although nobody knows exactly why this is so. Foods high in iodine, and therefore to be avoided, are iodized salt, kelp and other seaweeds, shellfish, and fast foods (machinery in fast food restaurants is disinfected with synthetic iodine, giving the foods prepared in it a high iodine level). On the other hand, many acne sufferers have no reaction to iodine. I must point out that iodine is essential to life and that even a mild deficiency can cause dangerous health problems. A thyroid gland inadequately supplied with iodine and Vitamin E can soon become so scarred that it will never again function properly. Some clinical studies suggest that organic iodine, in the form of kelp or kelp tablets, does not provoke pimples. Some authorities suggest that you experiment with iodine. They recommend that you try going without any iodine for two weeks, then try a few kelp tablets daily for another two weeks, and see if there are any dramatic outbreaks, or if they clear up when the iodine is discontinued. Nutrition expert Adelle Davis suggested taking a teaspoonful of kelp daily, or 325 milligrams of synthetic iodine once every week, obtained either from a tablet or from eight drops of tincture of iodine in a glass of water (tincture of iodine, she points out, is poisonous taken in quantity, but eight drops will not hurt you).

Chapter XI will give you the information you need on nutritional supplements. The basic program listed there contains all of the nutrients you need in the right amounts, although some can be boosted for acne. If they are boosted, they should be cut back when the problem is cleared up. A physician's or nutritionist's guidance is always helpful.

Increasing your Vitamin E intake to 400 units daily can help prevent scarring. Many doctors have recommended up to 100,000 units of Vitamin A daily, which seems to me not only excessive but possibly toxic if continued for a period of months or years. Furthermore, it has been shown that taking lecithin along with Vitamin A increases A's absorption to such an extent that 25,000 units are sufficient even in cases of severe illness. Two to four tablespoons of granular lecithin daily will also help your body metabolize fat. As for the B-vitamins, it will probably be best to take the antistress supplement two or three times a day, depending on which gives best results. Stick to the proportions of the antistress formula, and never exceed 50 milligrams each of B_1, B_2, and B_6.

While we're on the subject of the B-vitamins, boosting your biotin intake can be of great value, and if you happen to be in Canada or Europe, you can try the 5-milligram tablets that are regularly sold in drugstores there for oily skin and acne. The US RDA for biotin is 300 micrograms, which is the highest dosage available here. When taking large amounts of the Bs, always try to combine supplements with a natural food source high in them, such as liver, brewers' yeast, or, especially, wheat germ.

Before we leave the subject of Vitamin B, let me remind you that your intestines are a veritable factory for the synthesis of your own B-vitamins. Feed them lots of whole grains and vegetables, yogurt and bran, cut out the sugar, and you can be assured that they will be functioning at peak efficiency. Remember also that antibiotics, by killing off the intestinal bacteria that produce your own B-vitamins, increase your need for supplemental B-vitamins enormously, as well as for yogurt, bran, and sometimes Vitamin K and digestive enzymes. I firmly believe that antibiotics should be reserved for major illnesses where they could save your life; this is obviously impossible if you've grown immune by taking them for long periods of time.

There have also been many reports on the extraordinary value of zinc in treating acne. No one knows just why zinc is so helpful. Although clinical studies clearly show its ability to heal lesions of all kinds, they do not explain its apparent ability to *prevent* acne lesions in the first place. The US RDA for zinc is 15 milligrams, a level impossible to obtain on any normal diet, and deficiencies are widespread. Fifty to 100 milligrams daily is often recommended for acne, but it seems to me unnecessary to go above 50, especially when you are using the amino-acid-chelate form, which is better assimilated than the forms used in earlier studies. But by all means, here, as with any such experimentation with dosages, get your doctor's go-ahead first.

Finally, don't forget the unsaturated fatty acids, or Vitamin F, 15 grams of which should be taken daily, as indicated in the nutrition chapter. These acids are essential for normal fat metabolism, as well as metabolism of the oil-soluble vitamins. And acne is, after all, a disorder of fat-gland metabo-

lism. Unsaturated fats, yes; saturated fats and refined carbohydrates, no.

STRESS

At any age, someone with a normally dry or oily skin can be
subject to a sudden outbreak of blackheads or pimples. Sometimes this is due to a change in diet, or to some medication,
but often it is caused by stress, or nervous tension. Taking
one or more of the nutrients known for their tranquilizing
effect—calcium, magnesium, and Vitamin D—can be of
enormous help. Dr. Robert Atkins suggests that the B-vitamin inositol has an effect on the brain similar to that of a
moderate tranquilizer sedative. He found 650 milligrams to
be an effective daytime sedative, and 2,000 milligrams at
bedtime "a remarkable sleeping medication." He also reports
that Dr. Carl Pfeiffer, a noted authority on biochemical ab-
normalities in psychological disorders, has found the
2,000-milligram dosage effective in treating high blood
pressure. German research further indicates that both inositol and pantothenic acid, the B-vitamin most abundantly
supplied by the antistress formula, together have an influence both on the scalp, preventing dandruff and hair loss in
many cases, and on the skin, regulating sebaceous gland and
inflammatory changes, two factors of great importance in
dealing with pimples aggravated by stress.

It would be wonderful if we could avoid stress entirely, but
we can't. Stress can be caused by any number of emotional
and environmental factors, or it can be caused physically, by
illness or injury. Conversely, psychological stress often
causes severe physical illness, so it is not surprising that it
can aggravate cases of acne. Nutrition offers help in counteracting the effects of stress, and external care can do much to
relieve pimples caused by it.

If you are following the suggested routine for your skin type but are occasionally subject to pimples, you can deal with them as follows: continue to use the cleansing lotion as formulated for your skin type, since the acne cleansing lotion may be too strong. However, apply zinc oxide ointment to the affected areas after cleansing at night, and the antiseptic powder after shaving. You can also use the at-home mask for acne up to once a day, being careful to apply it only to affected areas, especially if you have dry skin. If you do have dry skin, don't apply a nourishing cream at night to the affected areas—use only zinc oxide ointment. Or you can dot each pimple with calamine lotion.

The occasional pimple can sometimes be more of a problem to extract than ordinary acne, especially if your skin is dry, because the pores are so small. One or two trips to a skin-care specialist (if you are not going to one regularly anyway) should be enough to take care of sporadic outbreaks. And be thankful that for you, unlike many adolescent *and* adult Americans, it's not a monthly, let alone weekly, routine.

SIX

AGING SKIN

N O, YOU CAN'T keep your skin from aging, but you can slow down the process considerably. There is no secret involved, nor is it a matter of artificially prolonging youth through camouflage or gimmickry. On the contrary, any man can—and should—keep his skin looking younger longer simply by learning how to take good care of it and using good common sense. The truth is that most men actually speed up the aging process by ignoring or mistreating their skin; improper care is the most significant factor in the deterioration of your skin, and with it, your looks. To understand why this is so, you'll need to know something about the aging process itself. Although there can be many secondary factors involved, there are three primary causes of aging skin: loss of moisture, loss of oil, and loss of elasticity. Let's take them one by one and see what can be done about each of them.

LOSS OF MOISTURE

The first sign of dehydration is a network of fine lines on the face and neck. At first these lines may be barely visible, but as time goes on, they grow deeper, larger, and more obvious. The expression lines around the eyes and the corners of the mouth, in particular, are more exaggerated than they would be in properly hydrated skin. The problem is that the skin simply isn't attracting or retaining water the way it used to. Research has shown, in fact, that a young person's skin contains about 13 percent water, while that of an older person may contain only about 7 percent. Scientists have recently isolated a substance called the Natural Moisturizing Factor, or NMF, which gives the skin its ability to trap and hold moisture. With age, the body manufactures less and less NMF. We don't know precisely what dietary factors influence the body's production of NMF, but we do know that the substance itself is composed largely of amino acids (the building blocks of protein), minerals, and carbohydrates, so it is safe to infer that a diet rich in these elements is important.

Still, since some decrease in the production of NMF is both natural and inevitable, our main concern is preserving the body's existing supply and losing as little moisture as possible. We know that NMF is water soluble and is easily destroyed by strong soaps and detergents. Quick-weight-loss diets should also be avoided, since they dehydrate the body's cells, making people who've lost weight too fast look not only thinner but much older. Environmental factors also cause dehydration: the sun, which dries out the epidermis, and the artificial heat or air conditioning most of us live with at home and in offices, shops, and factories.

If it's beginning to sound like your skin's moisture supply is constantly under siege, it is, but there are several things you can do to protect it against each of these dangers. Chemists working in skin-care research have designed synthetic reconstructions of NMF which are now being added to various skin-care products. Some of these can be helpful, but the expense involved in producing the synthetics is so great that only tiny amounts of them actually are used in these products. It has been discovered, however, that fructose, the kind of sugar found in honey and fruit, is one of the most important components of NMF. When applied externally, fructose binds itself to the skin's protein structure, providing a powerful moisturizing influence. When fructose has linked up with skin protein, it also resists being washed away by water and even, to some extent, by detergents. This is another instance of modern research validating popular folk wisdom: the fact is that honey applications have been popular for thousands of years. It is also interesting to note that a patent was recently issued for a new and very expensive hydrating complex based on fruit sugars, an idea that also occurred to the ancient Egyptians and which has probably been in use since prehistoric times. Because of the proven value of their fructose content, you will find honey, fruit, and vegetables included among the ingredients for the products I recommend, especially those for dehydrated skin.

LOSS OF OIL

As you'll recall from our original explanation of the workings of the skin, oil is necessary to keep your skin lubricated, to protect it from sun, wind, and other drying environmental factors, and to prevent the loss of moisture and NMF from the skin cells. Unfortunately, as you grow older, your oil glands slow down production and you can wind up with a serious oil shortage. Special massage techniques, as well as the extra cleansing treatments described in Chapter VIII, can do much to stimulate the oil glands. Massage performs a twofold function, since it can also help remove the tough film of dead cells and dirt that sometimes collects on apparently dry, dull skin, preventing oils from reaching the surface. Another way to keep the oil glands functioning is to be sure to include essential fatty acids in your diet, especially those found in vegetable oils, wheat germ, and nuts. External applications of vegetable oil, which penetrates very deeply into the skin, can also help, which is why vegetable oils are frequently included in skin creams. No matter what precautions you take, however, your oil glands are going to slow down to some extent as you age, and unless you have extremely oily skin to begin with, you will need to give yourself extra protection through the proper skin-care program.

Correct skin treatment can help compensate for insufficient oil production in several ways. Soaps, detergents, and high alcohol content astringents often strip lubricating oil from the skin. Eliminate these products and replace them with a good cleansing lotion and moisturizer or protective emulsion, and you will see an immediate improvement in your skin's texture. It is also important to use a rich eye cream, since, in adult skin, the area around the eye never produces enough oil.

LOSS OF ELASTICITY

Loss of oil and loss of moisture primarily affect the epidermis, creating superficial wrinkles. The worst problem of aging skin, however, is loss of elasticity, with its resulting sags, which begins in the dermis, the layer of skin just beneath the epidermis. In young skin, the dermis is full of a special protein, which forms many flexible, elastic fibers. As you grow older, this protein, called soluble collagen, becomes insoluble and the fibers lose their elasticity. Because they no longer have the strength to hold up the skin, the face begins to sag. To make matters worse, the weight of sagging forces the skin to produce more skin cells, forming bags and creases, especially in the areas of the eyes, neck, and jawline.

Good nutrition is essential to the preservation of the skin's collagen supply. We know that Vitamin C, calcium, and high quality protein, for instance, are particularly important, and a diet lacking in these nutrients will almost certainly speed up the deterioration of this crucial substance.

The single worst threat to your skin's collagen, however, is the sun. The whole mechanism of tanning, as you'll see in the chapter on that subject, is the skin's attempt to protect itself and its supply of collagen against damage by the sun's ultraviolet rays, not only because that damage can be severe, but because it is permanent and, to a large extent, irreversible. Moreover, the damage is cumulative, which is to say that deep tanning for only a week or two during every summer *will* hurt you eventually.

Unfortunately, the only way to avoid the destructive effects of ultraviolet rays is to avoid the rays themselves, either by staying out of the sun altogether, or by conscientiously using an effective sun block every time you are exposed. For many people, of course, the damage has already been done; in this case, you can alleviate the problem to some extent through facial exercises (and I'll provide a program of these in Chapter XII), which help tone the damaged tissue, and by sticking to a good diet.

Collagen, by the way, is sensitive to heat, as well as to ultraviolet rays. This is why I'm against the water-hot-as-you-can-stand-it shaving routine. You should avoid very hot showers and the steam baths at your local health club for the same reason: the heat not only dehydrates the skin but virtually "cooks" collagen as well, making it weaker and less elastic.

The treatments I have recommended to combat aging are, as you can see, primarily aimed at giving your face the same kind of protection against the environment afforded the rest of your body by clothing. It is, for the most part, a simple matter of adaptation: if the sun's rays are destructive, avoid the sun or provide your skin with a barrier against it; if artificial heating and air conditioning are drying your skin, get a humidifier; if your oil glands do not produce enough lubrication and protection from inside the body, give yourself that protection with products applied externally.

Your face does not get even the minimal cover-up a

woman's face gets from cosmetics (although it does have an advantage over women's skin in that it gets massaged every day when you shave); obviously, it is up to you to help your skin survive the wear and tear of the years.

Apart from these general changes, which are more or less symptomatic of all aging skin, there are two specific conditions you may have to deal with as you get older: couperose skin, or broken capillaries, and lentigo, or, as it's more commonly known, liver spots.

COUPEROSE SKIN

Couperose skin becomes visible as small, red, dilated veins, or masses of veins, just under the surface of the skin, usually on the nose and cheekbones, but sometimes all over the face. It often affects people whose skin is naturally dry, but it can happen to anybody. Men who spend a lot of time out of doors, exposed to extremes of weather, are particularly vulnerable.

At the onset of the problem, these veins may be barely visible, but if left untreated, they can spread and rapidly become more prominent. For this reason, it is important that you see a dermatologist at the first sign of them. In many cases, a doctor will be able to get rid of broken capillaries either by "sparking" them off with an electric needle, or by means of dry ice applications. Obviously, neither of these is a home remedy; they must always be performed by a competent professional. Still, there are certain ways to care for couperose skin at home, and certain things to know if you suspect you may be prone to it.

Couperose skin can be caused by internal or external factors: problems in the circulatory system, the intestines, or the liver; a vitamin deficiency, especially a deficiency of Vitamin C and its affiliate, Vitamin P (the bioflavinoids, rutin and hesperidin); or by constipation. Cigarettes and alcohol can also cause broken capillaries by interfering with proper circulation. In fact, because couperose skin is so often linked with general congestion and circulatory problems, it can, in some cases, function as an early warning sign of heart disease, another reason that any man, particularly a mature man, with this problem should consult a doctor immediately.

Among the external causes of couperose skin are any extremes of temperature: freezing winters, sweltering summers, wash water that is too hot or too cold, or the shock of alternating hot and cold water on the skin. Physical injuries can also involve the breaking of capillaries.

If you do have broken capillaries or a tendency toward them, you should be extremely careful of your diet. Eat lightly, avoiding alcohol altogether, and in general, staying away from hard to digest items such as fats, canned meats, and pickled, preserved, or highly spiced foods. Do eat fresh fruit and vegetables as much as possible. And get plenty of exercise, which will improve your all-over circulation.

Obviously, it is important to be gentle with your face. Avoid strong soaps and products with a high alcohol content, and rinse with water at room temperature. Use a protective cream whenever you are going to be exposed to the weather, and do not massage your face at all. Instead, use the masks recommended for your skin type (being careful, however, to avoid those containing brewers' yeast, which may overstimulate your skin).

There are also a number of natural ingredients you can add to your at-home mask which will help calm the angry red look of couperose skin. Among them are fresh apricot, cabbage, parsley, and orange juice, rose hip tea, and fresh green pepper juice with a few drops of honey added. Add enough of any of these to make a paste when combined with one tablespoon of the at-home mask.

LENTIGO (LIVER SPOTS)

While liver spots, as they are commonly called, are not, in themselves, as unattractive as some of the other problems that can affect your skin—acne, for instance, or even the broken capillaries we have just been discussing—they can be among the most psychologically painful because they are so generally associated with old age. Liver spots often affect fair-haired, fair-skinned people who spent a lot of time in the sun at some point in their lives. They show up most often on the back of the hands, the neck, and the face. Dermatologists can often remove liver spots with dry-ice treatments, or you can try bleaching them yourself by rubbing them with a little fresh lemon juice, applied directly or with a piece of cotton. Or use a tablespoon of lactic acid (available in drugstores) dissolved in two cups of water. You can also make a mask of one ounce of brewer's yeast and ten drops of twenty-volume peroxide, apply it to the liver spots, leave it on for five minutes, and rinse with water. If you do not see an improvement, try it again the following day, leaving it on an additional five minutes. You can increase the amount of time gradually, up to half an hour. Finally, you can add a small amount of plain yogurt to one tablespoon of at-home mask formula, to make a paste. Leave it on for the normal amount of time, then rinse with water. All of these preparations should, of course, be applied to a clean face.

Whether you have liver spots removed by a dermatologist or bleach them yourself at home, however, remember that they, like all pigmentation, will only disappear as long as you stay out of the sun. Renewed exposure will immediately bring them back again.

A FEW WORDS ABOUT PLASTIC SURGERY

Yes, more and more men are having face-lifts: one plastic surgeon friend of mine estimates that fully a third of his patients are male. And yes, the face-lift procedure is, by now, a straightforward, even a streamlined one; a face-lift can be given in the plastic surgeon's office in between four and five hours. And yes, a face-lift is safe and effective. It can completely remove the sagging around the jawline that we call jowls, the bags under the eyes, even the drooping *over* the eyes. It's just a matter of a few incisions, a few tucks, and a few stitches.

Why don't I sound more enthusiastic about a technique that's perfectly safe, within the financial reach of most men, and that does make a dramatic difference in personal appearance? There are three reasons.

The first is, a face-lift doesn't last. Even if you're very lucky and your face-lift "takes," you'll be right back where you started in ten years' time—in need of another face-lift. And if you're unlucky, you'll be in the same predicament after as short a time as *one* year. Face-lifts are temporary, and they are cosmetic.

Which brings us to the second reason I've never considered face-lifts the answer to all skin problems. Why address yourself to the symptom rather than the illness itself? Why spend money on the "pound of cure" when, for a fraction of its price, you can purchase the "ounce of prevention"? I mean, of course, that the battle against visible and unnecessary aging of the face begins not with a visit to the plastic surgeon when you're forty, but with proper at-home skin care (and appropriate behavior at the beach and on the ski slopes) from preadolescence. And certainly no later than when you turn twenty-one.

The third problem with a face-lift is that, while it can remove excess folds and sags, it is helpless when it comes to wrinkles—as blatant a sign of aging as jowls. Worse, a lift can't improve the *texture* of your skin. In fact, a lift may not have much effect at all on skin that has *bad* texture. As you know by now, only proper skin care can influence your skin's texture or retard wrinkling.

Now, don't misunderstand me. If you really do need a face-lift, and can afford one, by all means have it. Many men whose faces have been exposed to the sun and wind over a period of years, men who are construction workers, sportsmen, architects, woodsmen, and so forth, and who care about their appearance should consider it as a serious alternative; *they*'ve probably aged faster than any of their contemporaries. Likewise, men who work in television or movies or the theater have to be mindful of the potential desirability of a face-lift, as a kind of job insurance, if nothing else. And anybody who's come late to the principles of sound skin care may *need,* psychologically or physically, to look younger. Since he didn't invest in that ounce of prevention several years ago, he now has no choice but to purchase the pound of cure.

But even these men should realize that without proper *ongoing* skin care, without a thoroughgoing, custom-tailored skin-care regimen, no face-lift in the world is going to be truly effective. In fact, if you *do* decide you need to go through with a face-lift, it's more important than ever that you give your skin the kind of treatment it needs to revitalize the texture, improve the tone, and speed the healing process. Otherwise, you'll simply have succeeded in stretching some not particularly stretchable skin over the muscles and bones of your face. And, I can almost guarantee you, you'll be back under the plastic surgeon's scalpel in very short order indeed.

SEVEN

SHAVING

THE GROWTH of hair on the face is not only one of the things that separate men from boys, but also the major factor distinguishing male skin from female and, for too many men, good skin from bad. Shaving your face every day has an enormous impact on your skin and is, unfortunately, at the root of most specifically male skin problems. Shaving does have its advantages: by acting as a sort of minimassage, it boosts blood circulation and increases the skin's oxygen supply. But improper shaving techniques will, over a period of time, not only nullify these benefits, but do serious damage to even the healthiest skin. They will certainly make you look less than your best when you walk out of your door in the morning. Before outlining a program to safeguard your skin against shaving problems, I'd like to explain what goes wrong when most men shave, in order to help you understand why it might be necessary for you to change some of the products and procedures you've become accustomed to.

WHAT GOES WRONG

If you're like most men, you probably splash your face with lots of hot water, as hot as you can take it before shaving, because you've been led to believe it will give you a closer shave. This is simply not true. Lukewarm water works just as well, and a good cream applied before you shave does the job even better. Hot water is bad for any skin type. On a thick oily skin, it acts as a signal to the oil glands, telling them to pump out more oil than you need. On a dry skin, this stimulation of the oil glands is fine, but the overstimulation of blood circulation that accompanies it isn't. Dry skin capillaries tend to be very close to the skin's surface, and all that blood rushing to your face can, in time, cause these fragile blood vessels to expand to the breaking point, leading to ugly couperose skin.

Next, you apply shaving cream or soap to lubricate the beard area. In general, I have nothing against commercial shaving creams. Despite their chemical additives, most of them are reasonably safe, effective, convenient to use, and inexpensive. You should be aware, however, that some of them are extremely alkaline and will destroy your skin's protective acid barrier. This is not a problem as long as you follow a sensible *after*-shave routine, one that restores the acid barrier. If you're unsure about your shaving cream, however, suspect it is not doing the job or is irritating your skin, or if you simply dislike the idea of putting any chemicals on your face (as I do), you'll find the recipe for a safe, natural antiirritant shaving cream listed in the formulary. This is a rich emollient cream that wets the skin and beard thoroughly, swells the hairs for easier cutting, and provides a lubricating film to reduce microabrasions. The herbal extract contained in it is also soothing and antiseptic.

Then comes the shave itself. Because a blade—if you use a blade—pulls at each hair before it cuts, it naturally inflames the skin to some extent. And because the blade *is* a blade, it can't help but cause microabrasions, even if you're very careful. At best, these can hurt, and at worst, they can become infected. All this pulling and cutting gets worse, of course, the closer you shave. Which brings us to one of the worst mistakes men make in shaving: trying for the perfect close shave. This way of thinking is understandable, if misguided, since the advertisers of shaving products spend a lot of time and money convincing you of the importance of getting the closest possible shave. But let me say right now that shaving too close is definitely bad for your skin and is the main cause of many of your worst shaving problems. You're much better off aiming for a mild shave rather than a super-close one, and shaving again later in the day if necessary.

The typical routine ends with a quick rinse to get rid of remaining shaving cream or soap, followed, perhaps, by a splash of after-shave or cologne. Unfortunately, the rinse is almost never thorough enough to get rid of all traces of your pre-shave preparation, and a stubborn, extremely drying residue is left on the face. After-shaves and colognes make matters considerably worse. All of them contain large amounts of alcohol, which makes them extremely dehydrating, and often irritating, to the skin. And dehydration, as you know from our discussions of the skin and its functions, is one of the major causes of dull, flaky skin and premature wrinkling. Moreover, there is the additional risk of an allergic reaction to a fragrance or coloring agent; even though such reactions are rare, you should consider whether you are willing to court one.

That's what happens when most men shave. Now let's take a look at two important components of the shaving routine, your razor and blades, and then at two simple, sensible, no-nonsense shaving programs—one for manual, one for electric shavers—that will eliminate these daily hazards to your skin.

RAZORS AND BLADES

I think the new bonded razors, put out by a number of manufacturers, are best. I would advise you to try several different brands until you find one you're most comfortable with, whether it's single- or double-edged. Be sure to change blades at least once a week; sharpness makes a big difference in the quality of your shave and a sharp blade reduces not only razor pull, but the risk of ingrown hairs and blotchy skin as well. Obviously, fresh blades are doubly important for anyone with sensitive or blemished skin. And by the way, wiping the blade rather than rinsing it after use will merely dull it faster.

There are seven steps to the following shaving program. If it seems complicated or overlong, remember that you'll only have to spend two or three minutes on the actual shaving process itself, and you can be doing something else while you wait for the before/after shave emulsion to take effect.

SEVEN STEPS TO FOLLOW

(1) Five minutes before you're ready to shave, gently dab on about a tablespoon of your before/after shave emulsion (you'll find this product described more fully in the chapter on your skin type and directions for making it listed in the formulary), and spread it over the beard area. Be sure you allow the full preconditioning time, which is necessary to thoroughly soften and hydrate the whiskers.

(2) When you're ready to shave, rinse the face for one full minute with lukewarm water.

(3) Smooth a generous amount of your favorite shaving cream or the special antiirritant shaving cream over the beard area.

(4) Using a bonded blade, shave in long, smooth, slow strokes, always following the direction of hair growth (usually downwards). A light touch is what you're aiming for; the less you feel the blade against your skin, the better. Be especially careful around any areas that are broken out, especially on the neck. Try to shave around, rather than over, any existing pimples.

(5) Gently rinse off the cream with lukewarm water, splashing your face *thirty* times. This is necessary to remove drying residues.

(6) Apply your cleansing lotion. (Again, see the chapter on your skin type and the formulary for more details.) Saturate a piece of cotton with the lotion, then gently stroke over face and neck. The lotion is mildly antiseptic, but is also balanced to cool, calm, and hydrate the skin. Blot dry with a tissue.

(7) Again apply before/after shave emulsion, along with eye cream, if your face is dry, or apply to dry patches on oily or combination skin, as directed in the chapter on your skin type.

About Cuts

You shouldn't have any if you take your time, but of course, accidents can happen. Dab a little styptic lotion over the cut after step seven. The styptic lotion you'll find in the formulary is both mild and effective.

Irritation, Redness, and Pimples

If your skin is red and irritated after shaving, apply the aftershave corrective mask for fifteen minutes, as outlined in the chapter on your skin type. Why should it be irritated after all the trouble you've taken? Aside from simple carelessness, the most common cause is overzealousness in trying for too close a shave. It is also possible that your skin is simply very sensitive. If this is the case, I would advise you to switch to an electric shaver.

If you have little bumps or pimples around the shaving area, particularly on the neck, you should apply the aftershave mask to the trouble spots every day as a matter of course. The mask has a very rapid healing action, and daily applications should put an end to the problem within a few weeks.

ELECTRIC SHAVERS

It's no longer true that you can't get a close shave with an electric shaver; the new superthin foil-screen electrics such as the Braun Eltron do an excellent job, comparable to that of the old blade-type razors, but quicker and safer. I strongly recommend these new electrics for men with sensitive or problem skin. For one thing, they don't pull at whiskers the way manual razors do; for another, it takes fewer products, and fewer steps, to protect your skin than wet shaving does, which considerably reduces the possibility of irritation and abrasion. Although it's almost impossible to cut yourself with a good electric, you can give yourself razor burn, or micro-abrasions, by grinding away too hard or too intensively at the skin; again, the problem is a misguided pursuit of that elusive close shave. The shaving routine is, naturally, considerably shortened if you use an electric shaver.

(1) Start with the shave itself. I am against using commercial pre-electric shave lotions because of their strong de-hydrating effect. The purpose of these lotions is to reduce the slipperiness of the skin, a purpose they achieve by stripping the skin of precious natural oils. If your skin is too oily or moist to allow for a comfortable shave (this is really only a problem during the summer), simply dip a cotton ball in your cleansing lotion, apply it over the beard area, and blot it with a tissue. Wait three minutes for the lotion to dry completely, then shave. Your skin will be degreased, but not devastated. Don't stretch the skin in order to get a closer shave; this damages the facial muscles and paves the way for sags. Remember, better to shave twice a day than to overdo it once; the more so because touch-ups are so easy with an electric.

(2) When you've finished shaving, apply cleansing lotion, using the application method described above.

(3) Apply before/after shave emulsion and eye cream as directed in the chapter on your individual skin type.

Irritation

Should you notice a momentary skin irritation when you apply cleansing lotion directly after shaving, simply wait ten minutes, then apply it. This usually happens only if you have very sensitive skin, but any skin can overreact occasionally. If you are plagued by the chronic tiny pimples and whiteheads typical of shaving irritation, use the after-shave mask as often as you can—three times a week or even every day.

INGROWN HAIRS

This is a common condition that can vary in severity from a minor annoyance to a fairly serious infection requiring the help of a skin specialist. An ingrown hair is a curly hair that either reenters the skin or grows sideways *into* the skin, never quite emerging through the pore opening. If the problem is not serious, home treatment is simple: using a good pair of tweezers, gently straighten out the hair, pulling out the head so that the shaft comes only out of the original root. Do not, however, tweeze the hair out. Snip it off with a little pair of scissors, or a razor.

I can't emphasize enough the importance of gentleness in your shaving routine: gentleness in the products you use, gentleness in the way you manipulate your razor, gentleness in your overall attitude toward your skin, which will prevent you from hacking impatiently at your face and remind you instead to slow down, allow time for your pre-shave preparations to take effect and for your after-shave preparations to heal the skin again. Once you get used to this new way of approaching your skin and its morning ritual, I think you'll find the shaving process far less irritating, both mentally and physically, and a good deal more effective.

—————•—————

EIGHT

SPECIAL PROCEDURES
TO IMPROVE EVERY MAN'S SKIN

THERE ARE TIMES when your basic morning and night skin-care routine is simply not enough. No matter how disciplined you are about sticking to it, no matter how thorough you are in carrying it out, your skin occasionally needs the kind of *extra* stimulation and nourishment, plus a degree of *deep* cleansing, that routine daily attention can't provide, even under the best of circumstances. How often is "occasionally"? And how can you recognize those times? Those are not easy questions, and precise answers require a fairly detailed knowledge of your own skin, its type, habits, and weaknesses. But I can provide some guidelines.

If I had my way, I'd want every man, young or old, even if his skin is normal and functioning well, to have a professional facial once a month. The facial would provide him with a deep, rigorous cleansing and the skilled massage of experienced hands. Obviously, though, such a program is not always practical. For one thing, not everyone lives in an area where there are trained facialists. Second, not everybody wants to invest in a facial even twice a year, let alone once a month. And, most important, American business, and even American leisure, are not set up to accommodate a man's regular visits to a facial salon. Nor is the average American man geared to such a program psychologically. Eventually, I suspect, as men come to understand that their skin requires special care, and that providing such care does not constitute a threat to their masculinity, the situation will change. But for the present, I cannot censure any man who is hesitant about making monthly visits to a skin-care salon for the purpose of spending an hour with a facialist.

Many men do exactly that, of course, men who've found—or made—the time to take the best possible care of their skin. They *do* come to my salon on Manhattan's East Side, where they feel comfortable and not in danger of compromising their maleness. They make the investment of one hour and fifteen minutes and approximately thirty dollars once a month or once every two months to safeguard the vitality and health of their face. For those of you who've never visited a professional facial salon, I'd like to tell you what goes on at mine.

FACIAL AT PROFESSIONAL SALON

Before proper treatment can commence, your skin must be analyzed. On your first visit, I will give you a private consultation. I study your skin type and chart the course of the coming hour and fifteen minutes.

In a private room, as you relax in a reclining chair, you begin your facial with a thorough cleansing.

The second stage of the facial is massage, gentle and soothing, yet vitally stimulating to the blood circulation. Creams and moisturizers, prescribed for your skin type, are worked into your skin, penetrating the pores. I have worked out the movements of the massage from my knowledge of facial anatomy, and they will be explained by your operator. Do not hesitate to ask questions, for this is an educational experience.

Following the massage, your skin is once again cleansed; ozonated steam opens and disinfects the pores. Blackheads and whiteheads are removed. Soft brushing or superficial peeling removes dead cells. You are now ready for the masks.

Two masks are administered, chosen from the dozens of preparations I have scientifically blended. They may be made from jelly, wax, hops, or a variety of other natural ingredients, and their purpose may include smoothing the skin, calming inflammation, preventing wrinkles, removing dead cells, or hydration, depending on your particular needs. You are also instructed in the proper method of applying and removing masks so that you will be able to apply them yourself at home.

After your masks have been removed, I will again examine you and will discuss any problem areas.

We use no complicated machinery at my salon, and the preparations mentioned throughout are similar to the ones I've referred to in the body of this book and provided formulations for in the formulary. Now you can see that it is easy to give yourself an excellent, professional-quality facial in the privacy of your own home at a time that is convenient for you. And once you've realized how simple giving yourself a facial can be and how dramatic the results, it wouldn't surprise me if you undertook the whole process not once a month, but twice.

FACIAL AT HOME

In summary, the six basic steps of the facial are:

(1) Preparation, including basic cleansing
(2) Application of massage product
(3) Massage
(4) Steaming of the pores
(5) Superficial peeling (optional)
(6) Mask

That is the complete facial. There will be occasions when you'll have time to do just one or two of these procedures. But there is nothing like the *complete* facial, as I outline it here, to provide stimulation, nourishment, tightening, and cleansing—not to mention a pronounced sense of well-being. If you do undertake a complete facial, you must perform the steps in the order I gave them. Now, let me elaborate on each step—especially on the massage, which is easily the most complicated, and arguably the most important, one.

Cleansing

Basic cleansing of the face and neck is the first step. Begin with clean hands and nails, to avoid the spread of any bacteria. (You may also want to be newly shaved at this point, though I don't insist on it.) Then cleanse your face with your established cleansing lotion, downward, just as you do every morning and every evening of the month.

The second step is the application of your basic massage product to your clean face. Now, what, exactly, is a massage product? Well, that depends on your skin type. A man with dry skin should use a night cream, which is rich and nourishing. A man with dehydrated skin should use a combination of half night cream and half his accustomed moisturizer. Normal and combination skins should use a light mineral oil, which will only lubricate, not penetrate. Oily skins use only talcum powder. And what about the man who suffers from acne, pimples, eczema, or other open sores of one kind or another on the face? He mustn't massage at all, I am sorry to say. Manual manipulation of the facial skin could irritate the problem skin, overstimulate the sebaceous glands, *and* spread infection.

Applying the Massage Product

There is a seven-step sequence involved in the application of the massage cream or product. Trust me here. Though it all seems unnecessarily lengthy, it won't take as long to do it, once you're familiar with the motions, as it does to read about it here. Now, for the steps:

1. *The Neck:* Tilt your head slightly up. Hold all four fingers together, and make sure you use only the fingertips. Then, with the left hand, make one stroke on the left side of the neck, from the bottom, near the collarbone, up toward the jawbone. Follow with another stroke from the right hand along the same path. Repeat the same two movements on the right side of the neck, and in the center, right up over the Adam's apple and up to just below the chin.

2. *Chin to Temples:* With both hands making the same movement simultaneously on both sides of the face, place the four fingers—again held together—flat on the chin, and stroke up over the jawbone and out toward the temples. Repeat twice.

3. *The Upper Lip:* Starting at the outside corners of the upper lip, make four short strokes with the middle finger of each hand inward along the upper lip, so that the two fingers meet at the center.

4. *The Cheeks:* With both hands working first on one side of the face, then on the other, place the four fingers together on each side of the nose and stroke upward along it. Without lifting the fingers, smooth up over the eyebrows, across and out to the temples, and down to the outer corners of the eyes. Repeat three times.

5. *Eyes:* First, with the eyes closed, use the middle finger of each hand to make a few *very* gentle strokes down from the eyebrow through the center of the lid to the base of the eye. Then, with the eyes open, use the same finger of each hand to make comparably gentle strokes from the outer corner of the eye, across the under-eye area, to the inner corner.

6. *For Crow's-Feet:* Using the index and middle fingers of each hand, apply gentle "piano" movements (in which you tap the two fingers alternately, as if you were playing the piano), at the outside corners of the two eyes. Move up, then down. Don't stretch the skin or use too much pressure in this area; it's delicate.

7. *Forehead:* Hold the middle and ring fingers together. Using only their tips, make strokes from the eyebrows to the hairline, using first one hand and then the other.

That concludes the preparation of the face and neck for the massage itself. Dry, dehydrated, normal, and combination skin types will now be lubricated; oily skin types will have made sure excess oiliness was absorbed in the course of the massage. Now, as to the massage itself: I have the following remarks to make, which I hope you will read very, very carefully.

ABOUT THE MASSAGE

The word "massage" comes to us, most directly, from the French, but long before that there were similar words in other languages, including Portuguese, Latin, and Greek. These words had a common meaning—something roughly like "knead." Massage is a very old technique, used since ancient times to produce very specific changes in both the superficial and deep layers of facial skin, to help maintain the vigor of the skin muscles as well as the elasticity of the skin itself. If you'll forgive a bad pun, you really need to knead your face.

Facial massage techniques are both curative and preventive. If you're fifty and have never had a facial massage, you can't eliminate the wrinkles that you already have, but you can reduce their depth and severity; more important, you can help prevent the formation of new ones. If you're twenty, the age when the aging process begins in earnest, you'll probably be able to extend your wrinkle-free "youth" by a good ten or fifteen years. And it's not only wrinkles that are combated. Massage also acts against the folds (jowls are an example) caused by the widespread and premature relaxation of skin muscles and tissues.

What is the secret behind the facial massage? There is none, really, unless you consider human physiology a sequence of secrets. Massage creates a strong flow of blood through the tissues and stimulates the sebaceous glands, the secretions of which contribute to the maintaining of a desirable acid mantle on the skin. It creates better muscle tone, and promotes elasticity. It prevents the subcutaneous accumulation of oil deposits, while removing the superficial layer of dead cells. Finally, it decongests and relieves the redness of congested skin. (The only kind of skin *not* helped by massage is, as I mentioned earlier, that which is plagued by acne, eczema, or other open sores of any kind.)

Now, there are some things that massage clearly cannot do, and I feel it is my obligation to tell you exactly what they are. First, neither massage nor facial exercises (I'll supply some of these in the last chapter) can strengthen muscles that are already weakened by age. Neither can they in any way alter the contours of the face. And if they *could* rejuvenate and reshape facial muscles, they would, as techniques, be too intense and strong; I'd have to advise against them. Why? Well, they might damage the skin more than improve it. And, like body exercises, you'd have to maintain a *daily* routine, never missing so much as one day if you're to keep tightened muscles from sagging back to their "normal" state.

And what's the problem with daily massage, you might ask? It's simply too much of a good thing. Just as you shouldn't exert too much pressure in a facial massage (or, for that matter, any massage), for fear of doing harm to the muscles, so you shouldn't massage your face for more than five to ten minutes a day or more frequently than a couple of times a week. No matter how good your massage feels!

MASSAGE TECHNIQUE

One last word. Take the time now, at the outset, to learn the techniques precisely. Practice them. They're vital if your massage is to offer you all the benefits it's capable of conferring.

The facial massage begins with the forehead. Make sure that your hair is off your forehead, pulled back with a sweatband if necessary, and that you've applied all over your face the appropriate massage product, as I've discussed above. Now, you begin with the Zigzag Movement.

Zigzag Movement. With the middle fingers placed at points a and b, as in the accompanying diagram, move the fingers together in the direction indicated by the arrows. Then reverse directions. Make these movements across the entire breadth of forehead, then back again. Repeat the sequence as many as four times if the forehead is very lined.

Up-and-Down Movement. Cup each hand, holding the fingers closely together. With the tips of the fingers resting on the forehead, move one hand up, one hand down simultaneously, thereby creating friction. Move from one side of the forehead to the other. Repeat this sequence up to four times, if forehead is very lined.

Circles Under the Eyes. Place both middle fingers at the eyes' outer corners. Make three circles, very gently. Mov-

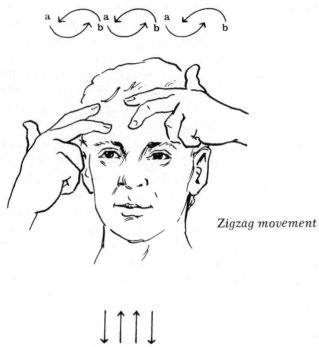

Zigzag movement

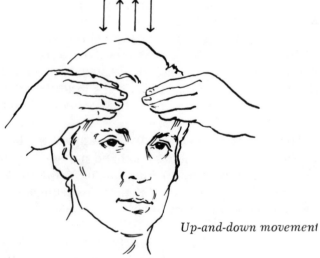

Up-and-down movement

ing to the middle of the under-eye area, make another three
circles. Moving to the inner corner, make yet another three
circles. Repeat the entire sequence three times.

Piano Massage. Tapping the four fingertips alternately in a very rapid movement, as if you were playing the
piano, move around the eyes in the direction of the arrows
three times. If you have any broken capillaries in this area
(most people do), repeat the sequence three times. Piano
movements should always be *extremely gentle.*

Circles on the Sides of the Nose. With the index finger
of each hand on the side of the nose, make four little circles
on the sides of the nose at points a, b, and c. At point c, after
you have made the circles, smooth up over the eyebrows,
across and out to the temples. Let your fingers rest on the
temples, d, for a second. Repeat two more times. If you have
blackheads on the nose, repeat the whole sequence two or
three times.

Piano Movements for the Entire Face. Using both
hands at the same time, make the same gentle piano movements all over the face and neck, from the forehead, moving
down gradually over the cheeks to the chin, under the jawbone, to the base of the neck. This sequence shouldn't last
more than thirty seconds or so.

However, if you have congested or blotchy skin, clogged
pores, or broken capillaries, repeat the sequence at least another three or four times, spending three to four minutes altogether.

Continue the movements all the way down to the shoul-
ders.

Mouth to Temples. This is a one-stroke movement.
Starting just under the nose, and using both hands at once,

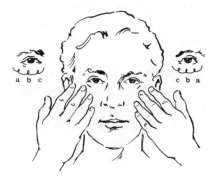

Circles under the eyes

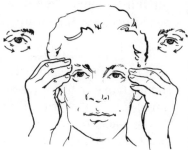

Piano massage

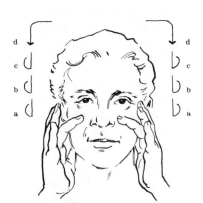

*Circles on the sides of
the nose*

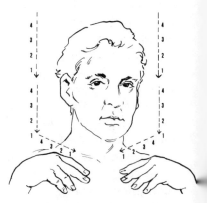

*Piano movements for the
entire face*

place the second fingers touching each other at point a, and the third fingers at point b. Stroke gently up toward the temples. Repeat a total of seven times.

Chin to Temples. With the middle fingers placed just over the jawbone, a, and the index fingers placed just under the jawbone, b, make five strokes along the jaw from chin to temples. If you see the first signs of a double chin, you may repeat this stroke up to twenty times. Alternate the strokes, first with the left and then with the right hand.

Nose-Mouth Fold to Temples. This is an elaborate movement, but it is important in treating the laugh lines that form from the corners of the mouth inward to the nose. With the second, third, and fourth fingers held *loosely* together, make three strokes from the corner of the mouth, lifting the corners of the mouth, up over the nose-mouth line and slightly out to the sides of the nose.

At the third stroke, continue up along the sides of the nose, to the eyebrows, and across and out to the temples. Rest your hands for a moment at the temples if you wish. Repeat the sequence three to six times; how many times depends on the severity of the laugh lines.

The Neck. Make a loosely cupped hand. Tilt the head back slightly and use the backs of your hands to alternately stroke from the throat line to the chin.

For Double Chin. Use the same alternating strokes of the cupped hands and the backs of the fingers.

(a) Tilt head up for half a dozen strokes under the chin. Then level head for another half dozen strokes.

(b) Pat under the chin with backs of cupped hands gently a dozen times.

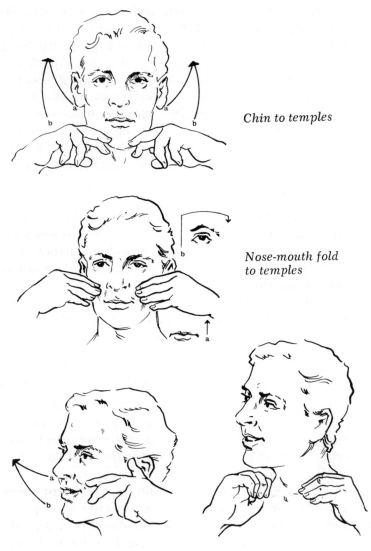

Chin to temples

*Nose-mouth fold
to temples*

Mouth to temples

The neck

The Tapping Massage. Starting on the neck, with the third and fourth fingers held together, tap with the fingertips very lightly. On the same spot, tap twice with the left hand and once with the right (or vice versa). Develop a quick 1-2-3 rhythm, with the emphasis on the first tap. Tap all over the neck, moving upward to the jawline, cheeks, and forehead. Do not tap around the eyes. (In the illustration, the numbers represent the sequence that is usually observed in a professional facial massage.) If the skin is very oily, tap very lightly and not too much. If the skin is dry, you may apply more pressure and tap for a longer time.

The Stroking Massage—to Complete the Massage. Use the same movements and sequence as you did when applying the massage cream, but more quickly and lightly. And for each step in the application massage, make five to ten times as many strokes as you did then.

The strokes should be very fast, but when you get to the forehead, you may reduce the pace, making long, gentle, slow strokes.

THE FACIAL STEAMING

After the massage, the rest of your at-home facial will seem a snap. That's not to say that the deep cleansing, the optional superficial peeling, and the applying of a mask aren't each important in their own way—only that the massage is the most elaborate step. And in a way, the most taxing.

The steaming procedure is, by contrast, an opportunity to relax. Its most important benefit is to bring the oily deposits deep in the pores to the surface of the skin. These deposits are then flushed away by the peeling and/or the mask. But before you do anything else, once again cleanse your face with cleansing lotion to remove any traces of cream, oil, or

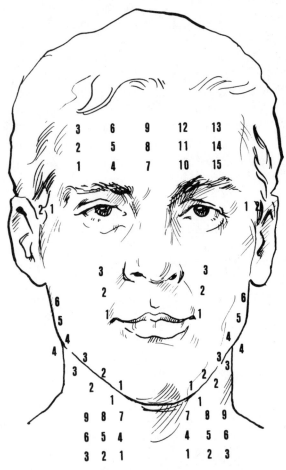

The tapping massage

talcum. Then be sure to apply some eye cream around your eyes, an area that can be irritated and even wrinkled by steam. If your eyes are very, very sensitive themselves, use a pair of eye shields, the kind you'd wear under a sun lamp. Now, once again, pull any hair that lies across your forehead *off* the forehead and secure it back with a sweatband. Your face should be totally exposed.

The first order of business: prepare the steam. To two quarts of water, add about a cup of chamomile flowers or three chamomile teabags. Heat in a good-sized pot (at least eight inches in diameter) until the water boils. Now, remove the pot from the heat, rest it on a tabletop or other flat surface, place your face over the pot (ten to twelve inches above it is best), and cover your head and, of course, the pot, with a bath towel. Steam for five to ten minutes, then pat your face dry. Tissue vitality and fresh, healthy pores are the benefits of the steaming process.

PEELINGS AND MASKS

As you know, the superficial peeling removes dead skin cells, aids blood circulation, and improves skin texture. You've already read in greater detail about the right one for you in the chapter dealing with your skin type; oily skins use cornmeal as the base for their peeling and all other skins use wheat bran. (The formulas are in the formulary.) The superficial peeling is optional here, as I have said; in any event it shouldn't be undertaken more than once or twice a month.

The mask is *not* optional. Every good facial should conclude with one, if not two, designed to correct specific skin conditions and shortcomings. There are dramatic, enjoyable, and unique benefits to be derived from masks in general. You will find them most helpful, not only at the end of the facial when they are essential, but whenever you have a few minutes to spare to upgrade, nourish, or "pick up" your complexion.

So much for the at-home facial. The whole procedure will take anywhere from twenty-five to forty-five minutes, depending on whether you include the superficial peeling, how

long you steam your face, the intensity of your massage program, and so on.

BRONZERS FOR MEN

Bronzers are makeup—not treatment—products. Most
men's bronzers now on the market contain moisturizers of
one sort or another, but while they do help the color absorb
into the skin more easily, and do afford the kind of protection
any moisturizer does against cold and dryness, the fact is
that you could wear the moisturizer without a bronzer in it.
In my opinion, that makes bronzers purely cosmetic. And
while I'm not opposed to cosmetics for anybody—men or
women—on a philosophical or aesthetic basis, I can't really
be enthusiastic about this category of cosmetics. Bronzers,
you see, contain alcohol, which can't help but be drying to
the skin. They also contain various dyes and chemicals that,
while not intrinsically harmful, can sometimes cause allergic
reactions. Why tempt fate?

Still, if you aspire to the air of vitality that a bronzer skill-
fully applied can achieve (I'll be the first to admit it), let me
tell you the best way to apply such a preparation. Begin with
a face that's been cleansed, toned, and moisturized according to the appropriate regimen. Yes, moisturize *before* applying even a bronzer that bills itself as containing "moisturizing ingredients" or the like; this assures an evenness of
application and, besides, you'll be using the moisturizer appropriate for your skin type, one to which your skin has
grown accustomed. *Then* take the bronzer, which is probably
in gel form in a plastic tube (sprays and sticks have been
largely discontinued), and squeeze a little onto your fingertips. Be careful, a little goes a long way. Now, whether you'll
want to apply the bronzer uniformly to your entire face and
perhaps even your neck, or whether you'll want to use it only
to emphasize *portions* of your face, is up to you. I favor the

latter approach, which highlights those parts of the face—brow, cheekbones, chin—that would be most affected by a day in the sun; no "tan" is ever completely uniform, after all. Whichever you choose, work swiftly to rub the gel into the various areas of the face, using small circular movements of the fingertips to do so. Even with all the moisturizer on your face, the coloring agents can splotch if allowed to remain piled up in a glob, rather than immediately rubbed in. Be precise, too—you're striving for a natural look. The whole purpose of bronzer would be defeated if it looked artificial—which is to say if it looked like makeup.

Now, let's pass from the face proper to the whole body, where skin problems of a different kind—a slightly different kind, that is—may await you.

·

NINE

THE WHOLE BODY

S O FAR, I have been talking almost exclusively about your face, about your complexion. True, I've also discussed the throat and neck—areas that, like the face itself, require specialized daily attention. Of course, they are the central concern in your shaving routine, too. But how about the rest of you: your back and chest, your arms and legs, your hands and feet, your scalp?

THE SKIN OF YOUR BODY

In this chapter, we'll take a close look at your whole body, its special daily challenges and dermatological needs. In the course of it, I'll have a few things to say about those two other forms of body covering—hair and nails—which, while less problematical than skin, can also cause trouble. Then, in the three chapters that follow, we'll consider the specific effects of the sun (and outdoor life in general), of nutrition, and of your "lifestyle" on the skin of your face and body.

Now, back to the question I posed a paragraph above. *Are* there differences between the skin of the face and the skin of the body? No, structurally, there are not. Like the face, the body is covered by the same highly stratified, multi-layered, blood-nourished, nerve-monitored organ that is your skin. Of course, there will be local variations. Not all human skin is endowed with oil glands, for instance, or with sweat glands, or with hair follicles. But those are very minor deviations, given the overriding unity of skin structure and function.

Moreover, they are no more extreme than the deviations that occur over the surface of the face itself. That is, not all areas of our face secrete oil, or sweat noticeably, or have hairs growing out of them. You don't shave your forehead, and you're not likely to get blackheads on your temples.

But there is one important difference between face skin and body skin, and it's a difference entirely of our own making: we protect the skin of our body with clothing from the sun, the wind, even to a degree from the pollutants present in big-city air. When it's cold, we wear gloves, but our faces are exposed to the harsh weather. In fact it's only in the course of sunbathing that the body comes in for anything like the kind of environmental battering that the face is expected to take, routinely. Moreover, we don't wash our bodies as often as we do our faces; they don't get nearly as dirty. And because we don't wash it as often, we don't dry it out as much: it is protected by whatever secretions of oil it can manage, as well as by layers of clothing. As a result, body skin tends not to dehydrate so readily or to age so quickly as the skin of the face.

Despite these safeguards, the skin of the body should not be abused. It deserves at least some reasonable minimum of care. Clothing doesn't protect it, for instance, from the drying effects of frigid winter air and of steam-heated offices and apartments. And you can complicate this situation by bathing too often during the winter months, when oil glands, slowed down by the cold, fail to secrete their usual amount of oil. Winter is also the time of year when the use of such popular health club amenities as the steamroom and the sauna are overdone. The skin of the body is capable of withstanding a considerable amount of seasonal variation and physical strain, and is *in general* less temperamental than that of face and neck, but it is not without its own sensitivities. Let's discuss bathing and showering first.

BATHING AND SHOWERING

In America particularly, but increasingly throughout the whole Western world, bathing—keeping clean, smelling good (or, more precisely, having no smell at all), combating even the most harmless germs—has become an obsession. It is, in my opinion, an unfortunate and an unnecessary one. For, while the face *must* be cleansed twice daily as a result of its oil-gland structure and of its lack of protection, the body hardly requires daily immersion in a bath of hot, soapy water or long sessions under a shower. Now, I'm not suggesting that people return to a policy of bathing only on Saturday night, or whenever it was that folklore decreed bathing be undertaken. But it is possible to keep clean with a well-deployed washcloth over the skin, reserving a full-fledged, no-holds-barred bath or shower only for every other, or even every third day. In the cold weather, many men would in fact profit from such a procedure—men who have dry, cracked, sensitive, flaking skin on their legs, elbows, sometimes even on their chests, and who wonder where it came from.

This condition comes from exactly the kind of dehydration that results from too long, too hot baths, utilizing too much soap, and taken too often. Here's what happens. You fill a tub full of water as hot as you can stand, climb in, and luxuriate for as long as you have time for. Meanwhile, you set about cleansing your body thoroughly with an alkaline soap, perhaps even a deodorant soap. Unfortunately, in the course of the cleansing, you strip the skin of all natural oils, thereby drying it. In the course of luxuriating, the heat of the water causes pores to fly open all over the body surface; that's all right, but they're going to remain open even after you've climbed out of the tub. And it's then that that supercrucial substance, simple moisture, is going to be lost, in significant quantity. The result: skin that's both dry *and* dehydrated.

What can you do about it? Of course, you don't want to give up bathing. In fact, I doubt that you'll even want to *consider* my suggestion that you refrain from daily bathing. The habit is too ingrained at this point, the feeling of psychological well-being that follows a morning shower or a before bed bath (or, alas, both) too familiar. But you can still cut down a bit. Begin by showering, rather than bathing, whenever possible; at least in a shower you're not totally immersed in water. Your skin can still breathe normally, at least to some degree, and pores won't have a need to open quite so wide to accommodate massive infusions of heat. But limit your showers (or, if you insist, your baths) to ten minutes, five if it's winter and your skin has already shown a tendency to become dry. And limit the water temperature, too: *don't* use water as hot as you can stand. That's harmful, no matter how good it makes you feel.

If you do bathe, make use of a bath oil. There are a number of good commercial products on the market, many of them reasonably priced. If you're of an economical turn of mind, even simple mineral or vegetable (sesame) oil will do the trick, perhaps scented with a few drops of a favorite cologne or after-shave; I recommend about a tablespoon per bath. A slightly more elaborate plan involves making up your own bath oil. Here's a foolproof formula that should provide enough oil for even very dry skin:

> 1 teaspoon vegetable oil
> 4 ounces witch hazel
> 1 pint water

Shake well, though, as the oil will separate rapidly out of the water. Even better, incidentally, is wheat germ, peanut, or safflower oil. Whichever you choose, add the resulting mixture to your bath, then stir the water around vigorously.

Even more important than using a rich, dispersible oil, in

my opinion, is *not* using a harsh, over-alkaline soap. This is true for every man, but it is especially true for men whose skin is susceptible to wintertime dryness. Now, if you require the extra protection of a deodorant soap, you'll have to be cagey about it. I recommend using the deodorant soap last, when it will have the least possible time to remain in contact with your skin, and I recommend using it only on those parts of the body—armpits, groin, feet—that really require it. For the rest of you, I propose an acid-balanced, emollient soap, to be used before the deodorant soap. You'll find recipes for two superrich soaps in the formulary; otherwise, a mild, commercially manufactured soap like Ivory or Neutrogena should present a minimum of problems. If dryness continues, despite bath oil and superrich soap, you can use a vinegar- or lemon-juice based lotion as a post-bathing rinse; just combine a tablespoon of either liquid with a quart of water, and pour slowly over the body to combat alkalinity.

Of course, after your bath or shower, make full use of a moisturizer or body lotion to counteract dehydration. It will help seal up those open pores, thus locking in moisture; it also soothes sensitive or weather-irritated skin, just as it does after a day on the beach. (I'll have more to say on the subject of moisturizers for the body, as opposed to the face, in the chapter on sun, which follows immediately.)

So much for bathing. I hope I've at least made you think twice about overdoing it, and provided some antidotes to its excesses. Now it's time to take a closer look at two related whole-body procedures, equally traditional but not nearly so essential—saunas and steam baths.

SAUNAS AND STEAM BATHS

The sauna is a Finnish innovation, and of the two, the one currently with the most vocal supporters. It makes use of high heat (between 180° and 190° F.) and low humidity (10 percent or even lower) to relax muscles and tranquilize the nervous system. It also raises body temperature, and may improve circulation. Claims have been made, as well, for sauna's eliminating body poisons, curing and preventing colds, and clearing up skin ailments and blemishes. These last seem doubtful, although it *is* true that such an exaggerated level of heat can benefit dry skin by stimulating its largely inactive oil glands to put out more than they otherwise would; of course, you shouldn't stint on moisturizer afterwards, for the same reason you don't after your bath. Oily skins may be *over*stimulated by such massive doses of heat and, conversely, sfor them a cleansing lotion or a mask should be used immediately after a sauna to remove excess oil from the skin surface; the mask will additionally help tighten the pores, which tend to enlarge in the sauna process. And because sauna will also stimulate the oil glands of the back, where acne can form as readily as on the face, oily-skinned men will want to use an astringent there—and anywhere else where acne and excessive oiliness are a problem. Beginners, by the way, should spend no more than eight to ten minutes in the sauna; maximum time for the veteran sauna user is fifteen minutes. And no one should use a sauna when under the influence of alcohol or narcotics, or when he's taken antihistamines, tranquilizers, vasoconstrictors, vasodilators, stimulants, or hypnotics. (Elderly people and those who suffer from diabetes, heart disease, or high blood pressure should avoid saunas altogether.)

The steam bath—also known as the Turkish bath—makes use of considerably lower temperatures, generally between 110° and 130° F. But because the air is so moist, it feels every bit as hot as the sauna. (It's like a day that's hot *and* humid causing much more pronounced discomfort than one that's merely hot.) Because of the high humidity, the sweat cannot evaporate and cannot have a cooling effect on the body. As a result, body temperatures soar, even more than in a sauna. Many experts question the safety of steam baths for this reason, even while accepting sauna. I'm not against steam *or* sauna, taken in moderation by men who are otherwise healthy, any more than I'm against a day at the beach. For one thing, steam baths are less likely to dehydrate the skin than saunas, although you still sweat a great deal, and lose critical body water, which must be replenished; that means using the same moisturizing routine afterward as we've discussed. Steam baths probably should be avoided in favor of sauna (if you *must* have some "intense heat" experience) by anyone whose skin is extremely oily. With all that sweat (which can't evaporate, as in a sauna), there is a risk of clogged pores.

Skin Tone

Before we leave the subject of steam baths and saunas, let me remind you of a subject we discussed earlier, with reference to the face. I refer to "tone," the elasticity and suppleness of the skin, so important to a youthful and healthy appearance. Tone is a complex quality, and derives from many different variables: everything from the number and placement of fat cells, to the blood and its subcutaneous circulation rhythms, to simple muscle strength and conditioning. Yes, some people just naturally have better skin tone than others, just as some people naturally have thicker hair or bigger bones. And there's only so much a man who has poor skin tone can do about it. One thing he definitely can do, though, is not overexpose himself to any form of heat, whether in a steam bath, a sauna, or stretched out on a beach. Such extreme and direct heat first brings about dehydration, then breaks down collagen. The result is a skin that's flabby, both on the face and all over the body. That means that you must keep your steam and sauna sessions within the recommended limits of time and temperature (health clubs and spas are fairly careful about this), and that, in the sun, you protect yourself with a lotion containing a sun-screening agent. Much more on the last in the next chapter.

I hope it's second nature to you by now to apply moisturizer—generously—after any exposure to heat. You *must* counter the effects of the inevitable dehydration immediately after showering off the sweat (and perhaps the salt and sand) from your body. Cover your whole body with a good, light moisturizer—a nongreasy one, too—like the one for which I provide a formula in the back of the book. That way, you'll stand a chance of slowing down the loss of skin tone, which, more than any other single factor, can make a man seem prematurely old.

EXERCISE AND MASSAGE

Exercise and massage are also valuable weapons in your ongoing war to maintain body skin tone. (Because the skin of your face isn't attached by muscles to the bones underlying it, exercise is less effective there.) The stretching and the strengthening that a good exercise program provides, together with the enhanced blood circulation produced by exercise, all aid tone—and can sometimes even add it, over the months and years. Likewise, massage can help tone the skin, not by strengthening muscles (it has absolutely no effect on muscle strength or flexibility), but by increasing the superficial blood circulation, which results in a stepped-up supply of oxygen to the skin. Needless to say, massage also confers real psychological benefits. But, as with sauna and steam bath, don't overdo; once a week is a sensible schedule, unless you've just lost a great deal of weight and have "loose" skin, in which case twice a week might be a good investment.

However, as I've already said very clearly in this book, neither exercise nor massage will do a thing for skin *texture*. That's solely a matter of conscientious daily care.

DEODORANTS AND ANTIPERSPIRANTS

No American man has to be sold on the idea of a fresh-smelling body, not just immediately after a bath or shower, but for the duration of his day. And that is, clearly, a function of deodorants and antiperspirants. Not everyone, however, understands exactly what these drugstore and supermarket products do. Let's begin by defining the difference between deodorants and antiperspirants. Deodorants contain chemicals (in an almost limitless variety) that kill bacteria. Antiperspirants, on the other hand, contain an aluminum salt (most often it's aluminum chlorohydrate) which inhibits both the manufacture and the flow of sweat. Antiperspirants alter a bodily process *and* attempt to nip the perspiration problem in the bud, before it's really surfaced. Deodorants allow the sweat to flow freely; they simply prevent the growth of bacteria. And since it's the by-products of bacterial metabolism that cause the odor associated with perspiration, not the perspiration itself, deodorants do an acceptable job of controlling odor, at least for most of us. If you wash with an antibacterial deodorant soap, at least under your arms (and I'll be the first to admit that they're generally harsh), you may not require a deodorant or an antiperspirant.

Your needs are determined, you see, not only by how much you sweat, but also by *why* you're sweating. Basically, there are two different kinds of perspiration: normal and nervous. They're both secreted through the same sweat glands and funneled through the same skin pores, but they're chemically different. Normal perspiration occurs constantly all over the body, the result of the body's having to cool itself down (evaporation is, after all, a cooling process) and get rid of certain waste products. Unless you've really overexerted yourself, whether by staying too long in the sun or playing too hard at tennis, this kind of sweat is virtually odorless. Nervous perspiration, on the other hand, is a neural response to certain mental states—tension and anxiety, for the most part—and it's fairly rigidly localized—in the armpits, the soles of the feet, and the palms of the hands. Nervous perspiration can combine tellingly with bacteria to cause body odor.

I bet you're expecting me to provide you with a formula for a homemade, all-natural deodorant. Well, I have no intention of doing so. Almost all of the deodorants and antiperspirants on the market are good, serviceable products that you couldn't really make any better—or any more cheaply— yourself. These commercial preparations come in various forms, of course, such as sticks, sprays, pumps, roll-ons, even pads and powders. And they vary considerably in strength; you'll have to assess the extent of your odor problem, if any, and act accordingly. Most important to keep in mind, though, is the fact that odor is the result not of simple sweat, but of that relatively innocent, innocuous sweat combining with bacteria. The most important thing you can do to combat a serious odor problem is to prevent the bacteria from acting on the sweat. You'll have a head start if you keep your underarms, your groin, and the soles of your feet clean.

While I have not offered a deodorant formula, I do want to take this opportunity to talk to any man whose palms or soles sweat excessively as a result of nervousness or, perhaps, of a simple superabundance of sweat glands in those regions. I recommend that you consider dusting the soles of your feet (between the toes, too) with a talc every morning, the palms of your hands whenever necessary, and certainly after each washing. You'll find a very useful talc in the formulary. The zinc oxide it contains acts to inhibit sweating as much as the aluminum salt in an antiperspirant does, and should take care of this particular problem.

HANDS AND FEET—AND NAILS

Hands and feet can be problems in other ways, too. Because the hands are not equipped with oil glands, and because they tend to be exposed to the environment more than other parts of the body, they can become very, very dry in winter. In the formulary, I give the recipe for a very rich hand cream that you can make yourself. And though I call it a hand cream, it's just as good for elbows, heels, even dry legs as it is for hands. If your hands are very chapped or very dry, apply the cream abundantly before going to bed. Men who do heavy work, a great deal of outdoor work, or who work around water will find such a treatment especially beneficial.

I don't have very much to say about manicures and pedicures—or about the nails in general. Obviously, the state of your fingernails says a great deal about your health, your profession, and your self-respect. But few men want to take the time to administer even a biweekly "professional" manicure, or are willing to seek out a manicurist. I suggest only that you keep your nails clean, clipped short, and free of hangnails and rough edges (the last by filing); the cuticles should be pushed back with as blunt an instrument as possible, and clipped away whenever they have overgrown. Toenails do, however, pose one additional problem—that of ingrownness. Here, the trick is to keep the nails short and trimmed straight across, *not* curved to approximate the shape of the toe. If you do have an ingrown nail, try slipping a tiny bit of rolled cotton under the edge that is pushing against the toe; this will not only relieve the pressure, but help to direct the nail in a more healthy, outward growth. Of course, any seriously ingrown nail requires the attention of a chiropodist.

Corns and Calluses

Corns are most often the result of ill-fitting shoes, calluses of simple wear and tear. Plasters and other commercially available products for the removal of corns are as good a suggestion as I can make, short of seeing the chiropodist. Calluses, which can build up and become painful as well as unsightly, are best treated by a vigorous rubbing with a pumice stone or even a rough cloth before they become hard and thickened. Let me close this discussion of hands and feet with a recommendation that you treat your hardworking, shock-absorbing, skeletally complex feet to an occasional footbath. Try soaking them in warm water to which you've added half a cup of sea salt or white vinegar. That's a simple and relaxing reward for them—and, indirectly, for the rest of you—at the end of a long day.

HAIR AND SCALP

I've deliberately saved the topic I suspect you are most interested in for last. I refer to your hair and scalp. Hair is, of all the different parts of your body, the only one that you can redesign, can cause to say something about who you are, at a whim. That's not a responsibility, mind you, but it is a wonderful option. Naturally, every man who wants to alter or maintain his image wants to have his hair in the best shape possible. And hair does take quite a beating. Fortunately, unlike skin, it's dead, or at least that part of it visible to the naked eye is; once it pokes its way through the scalp it's ceased, you see, to receive nourishment or sensation from the circulatory and nervous systems, respectively. But even though hair is dead, technically, it shouldn't—and needn't—appear lifeless. In the next few paragraphs, I'll tell you why.

As far as I'm concerned, the scalp is the only place to start.

The most important part of hair care is good scalp care, precisely because the scalp contains the hair roots and growth cells. These growth cells are continually growing hair, which they then push out through the hair follicle; at that point they'll usually rest for a while. At any given time, roughly 100,000 scalp cells—at least that number on the healthy head of a healthy man—are alternating between growing, pushing, and resting. Hairs are constantly being grown. And they're just as constantly being shed; in an average day, between fifty and a hundred will give up the ghost and fall out. That shouldn't alarm you, however. If they *didn't* fall out, there'd be no room for the new hairs currently under production and your hair would really be unmanageable.

Now, those hairs you see growing out of your scalp—perhaps in great profusion, perhaps all too few—require careful handling, even though they're dead. For one thing, they can't regenerate or rejuvenate themselves after damage. For another, they're fairly fragile, susceptible to heat, dryness, chemicals, and simple wear and tear. Blow driers can, as you probably know, have an especially deleterious effect on hair; always keep your hand-held drier (if you really must use one) twelve inches from your head, using low and medium heats whenever possible, even though that may mean a few extra minutes of drying time. Likewise, be wary of too much sun—whether on the beach, the tennis court, or the ski slope. Detergent shampoos and excessive amounts of hair spray can also take their toll. And while few men experiment with curl and color, those who do should be mindful that they are chemically altering the composition of their hair: dyeing, tinting, waving, and straightening are all very hard on the hair. While you *can* undertake any and all of them at home, there's a good argument for entrusting any of those processes to a trained professional. In any event, try to select a color, or a degree of curl, that doesn't have to be repeated too often.

I am not a hair stylist by profession, nor have I ever had remotely the same interest in hair, aesthetically and clinically, that I've had in skin. I tell you this so that you won't expect styling tips or know-how from me in these pages. I do, however, have an attitude, a philosophy, about hair. I think hair should look clean, healthy, and natural, and that a hair style should reflect all these qualities.

Of course, there are the same conditions—and problems—of dry and oily in the scalp as there are in the skin. And they can seriously interfere with the health of the scalp and appearance of the hair.

Oily Hair

Oily hair tends to be greasy hair. It also tends to be dirty hair, because dirt, soot, and the like adhere to the oily surface much more readily than they do to a dry one. Anyone with oily hair *must* shampoo at least once a week; some men will probably be happier shampooing every other day, especially if they live in big cities, where the air is often thick with dirt and pollutants. I do not have a formula for an oily hair shampoo to give you, but I will suggest that you use a commercial shampoo especially made for oily hair. You may have to experiment a bit to find the one that leaves your hair most manageable; you're not alone, though, as everyone must proceed by trial and error when choosing a shampoo for the first time. As for a conditioning rinse, there I can be of some help. Simply mix between one and two tablespoons of fresh lemon or grapefruit juice in one cup of warm water. You don't even have to rinse this mixture out. It will leave your hair manageable and shiny; it will also help restore the scalp's natural acid balance, which is disrupted by the alkalinity of any shampoo strong enough to be effective against oiliness.

Dry Hair

Dry hair is the result of dry scalp; lusterlessness and a "flyaway" tendency are the inevitable outcome. Because your scalp is so lacking in oils, you really shouldn't use soap on it at all. Instead, use an egg-yolk based shampoo. Beat two egg yolks and combine with one pint of water; shampoo onto the scalp and work through the hair. Then rinse well with lukewarm water and, to ensure manageability, add a little vinegar (a tablespoonful should do) to the final pint of rinse water. If extra lubrication is required, half a cup of beer (let it stand for a little while first) or an egg white (saved from one of the yolks you shampooed with) added to the final rinse can also work wonders. A brilliantine cream afterwards will both lubricate the scalp through the day and control any unruly hair strands.

Dandruff

Dandruff is the third basic scalp problem that many men suffer from. I don't have to tell you how unsightly it is; it can also be uncomfortable, itchy, sensitive. Excessive hair falling can result, which, while never permanent, is often alarming. Unfortunately, dandruff, though a seemingly simple disease, is still a poorly understood one. It can be hereditary. It can result from a malfunctioning of the hormones, of the thyroid and adrenal glands, or of the scalp itself. An irregular metabolism can exacerbate, and perhaps even cause, dandruff, as can certain nervous conditions, certain kinds of tension and anxiety. Dandruff may also be caused by an insufficiency of Vitamins A, B-complex, and E. Sometimes dandruff flakes are large, oily, and yellow; sometimes they're minute, dry, and powdery. I wish I could tell you that there is an easy way out of dandruff, but there isn't. A certain kind of dandruff shampoo may work for you, but not for a fellow sufferer, and vice versa. Sometimes alternating medicated shampoos containing different active ingredients, using one on, say, Monday, the other on Thursday, will turn the tide. Try it and see. But if you have no real luck with commercially available shampoos, or if your condition is advanced and/or pronounced, my best advice is to see a dermatologist. Dandruff is, after all, a disease—not, like oiliness and dryness, a mere tendency on the part of the scalp.

Scalp Massage

Almost all scalps—dry, oily, even that rare "normal" variety, as well as some dandruff-ridden ones—will profit from regular massage. In fact, I can think of few things as good for your scalp as a five- to ten-minute massage before shampooing. Like a face or body massage, the scalp massage stimulates the blood circulation, as well as the sebaceous glands, decongests, and encourages mobility and elasticity of the skin. You should massage when the hair is dry and, as I've said, before your shampoo; that way oily scalps will be able to wash away the oil secretion that will result from the massage itself. Also, make sure, before beginning, that your nails are cut and filed and your hands clean.

There are four steps to the scalp massage:

(1) Starting with the forehead, work to the top of the head, moving in small, circular motions. Use both hands at once, working with the fingertips from the forehead's center to the temples. At the temples, lift the fingertips and return to the center of the forehead. Repeat four or five times.

(2) Now apply the fingers of one hand to the forehead, those of the other to the back of the head. The fingers should be fixed on the scalp in one spot; apply pressure, and move the fingers up and down. Repeat five or six times, changing the hands' position so that the entire front and back areas are covered.

(3) Repeat the movement, but with the hands and fingers above the two ears. Use a circular motion to the right, then to the left. Repeat five or six times.

(4) Now, using the tips of both sets of fingers, begin at the back neck muscles and slide your hands up and forward, exerting firm pressure, until you traverse the entire scalp and arrive at the forehead. Repeat vigorously five or six times, slowing down at the end.

After the massage, brush your hair energetically with a hard-bristle brush, in all directions. You are both stimulating the scalp and lubricating the hair shafts by bringing oils from the scalp down their lengths. (If your scalp is oily, don't brush too much.) If your hair is dry, brush as much as you want— but not overenthusiastically, as you may break brittle strands. You are now ready to shampoo.

Baldness

And what about baldness? Is there some magical cure, dermatological or otherwise, for this almost exclusively male "failing"? I'm afraid not—but then you knew there wasn't all along. I'm talking, of course, about normal, hereditary male pattern baldness. Most other types of baldness can be corrected by a physician who specializes in scalp diseases. You can, of course, camouflage the problem, with anything from hair transplants, implants, reweaving, and so on (frankly, I'm confused by the plethora of new, and often painful and costly, methods for the artificial replacement of hair), to the simple toupee. But you can't, at present, *correct* it, and anyone who says you can, whether with vitamins, massage, or prayer, is misleading you. (There is some evidence that massage will slow baldness down, before it has actually run its course, but even this is at best buying time.) My advice to you is as an aesthetician rather than a clinician. Simply live with the baldness. Don't call attention to it, for instance, by combing a few long strands of hair over the bald spot. Don't bemoan it. You may find it both practical and appealing to get a short haircut, in fact, which will minimize the discrepancy between bald spot and surrounding areas of normal hair growth. You may even want to grow a mustache to divert attention from your head to your face. But here, as with most aspects of male grooming, natural, easy, and unassuming is best. If you don't appear to be living in the shadow of your baldness, nobody else will think very much about it.

———•———

TEN

YOUR SKIN AND THE SUN

W HAT COULD be friendlier than a sunny day, more relaxing than an afternoon at the beach, or more potent a symbol of health and vitality than a glowing tan? And yet, from the point of view of skin care, the sun has lately been shown to be a villain. We've always understood that too much sun will cause a sunburn, but only recently have scientists proved that redness and blisters are, in fact, the least of our worries. Sunburn pain may be intense, but it is nothing compared with the three kinds of skin cancer that overexposure to the sun can, over the years, give rise to. Excessive exposure to the sun can also cause premature aging—dehydration, wrinkles, and thickened, leathery looking skin.

I am not going to warn you never to go outside again on a bright summer day, for there are both physiological and psychological benefits to be obtained from sunshine. I am aware that because of the enormous cachet of a good tan, you might decide to ignore my suggestion and continue to "take your chances" at the beach. But I do want to explain just how the tanning process works so that you understand why careless tanning is so harmful to your skin, and why it is absolutely crucial for you to begin to take a *defensive position* against the distant, deceptive, and ultimately dangerous sun.

SKIN COLOR AS A STATUS SYMBOL

Before I begin, however, I'd like to put this tanning business in perspective a bit, by reminding you that, until fairly recently, bronzed skin was not the status symbol it is today. The Greeks may have admired a golden tan, but from ancient times until the 1920s, tans had about as much prestige as calluses. They immediately branded one a member of the laboring class—somebody who worked outside smoothing roads or picking apples or pitching hay. It was the laborers who changed color with the seasons while the leisurely, the affluent, the enviable, lived life indoors or under broad-brimmed Panamas, maintaining year round their smooth white skin. Pale skin became, over the centuries, one of the first status symbols, and even the yellow and brown races came to characterize their most beautiful women as "white as alabaster." And by staying out of the sun, royalty distinguished itself from the dark, field-working peasants; veins noticeable through the paleness, far from being a disadvantage, lent credence to the ideal of blue-bloodedness. It was not until industrialization gave rise to the factory system and deemphasized agriculture that menial labor moved indoors and pallor ceased to be the exclusive hallmark of the upper classes. Medical science discovered that without exposure to ultraviolet radiation (of which the sun is our only natural source) and in the absence of a diet rich in Vitamin D, rickets developed.

SUNBATHING

In the Twenties, doctors began prescribing sunbathing as a specific treatment for tuberculosis. A definite health and vitality advantage began to be gained by wealthy Europeans and Americans who embraced the new sun-drenched outdoor life. For the last fifty years, sunning has enjoyed increasing popularity not only on the beach, but by the pool and on the tennis courts, slopes, and trails. Witness the growth of the suntan lotion industry, which, since 1928, the year the first lotion was sold in a drugstore, has grown to an $80 million a year industry. But suntans, like pallor, are to a large extent an expression of the current fashion. Unrestrained, unthinking, and largely unprotected tanning has been the rage for a little over fifty years, and while no one is about to go back to the age of Panamas and parasols, it is not out of the question, now that the research is in, and we are beginning to see the disastrous results of overtanning on preceding generations, that we begin to adopt a somewhat more cautious approach to our time in the sun.

ULTRAVIOLET RAYS

The sun's ultraviolet rays—those responsible for both tanning and burning your skin—can reach you virtually anywhere at virtually any time—summer or winter, on the beach or the mountaintop, through clouds, under water, or even just reflected off the windows of an office building. These rays do confer certain benefits: their drying effects are a boon to both extremely oily and acned skin, and they do help your body synthesize Vitamin D to some extent. Nevertheless, more or less constant exposure puts a severe strain on all other skin types, and on those areas of oily or acned skin (such as the eye area) that do not produce excess oil. You should be familiar with how the sun acts on the skin in order to know when, where, and what kind of precautions are necessary for your particular lifestyle and skin.

THE TANNING PROCESS

The whole mechanism of tanning is designed to protect your skin and your internal organs from constant bombardment by the sun's ultraviolet rays. The body's chief defense against these rays is the melanin which was described in some detail in the chapter on black skin. When the skin is exposed to the sun, the special cells that produce melanin produce even more of it, and migrate slowly up to the surface of the skin, flattening out and overlapping to form a shield as they go. Once large quantities of melanin are evenly distributed in the tough outer layer of the epidermis, they protect the skin by absorbing and neutralizing the most damaging of the incoming ultraviolet rays. Not only does this allow you to stay out in the sun for longer periods of time without burning, but it also provides your skin with the color that is generally recognized as a tan. The existing melanin will stay in place until it is sloughed off naturally along with the rest of this dead outer layer of skin cells—a process accelerated considerably and somewhat dangerously by peeling. If exposure to the sun continues, the body must quickly send up a new front line of melanin to ward off further rays.

As you can see, the problem is largely one of allowing your skin enough time to produce its own protective forces and get them into place. This is why dermatologists and skin-care specialists make such a fuss about tanning *slowly;* unless you have black skin, it takes time for your body to manufacture and distribute its protective pigment. In the interim, your skin and its entire metabolism are being exposed to extremely harmful radiation. I do not want to sound like an alarmist but let me assure you I am not exaggerating; the effects of long or repeated periods of unprotected sunning are, quite simply, disastrous. What's even worse, the disaster is cumulative. Your skin "remembers" every minute you ever spent in the sun, and while the effects of a bad sunburn may seem to be only temporary, the true extent of the damage done will only begin to show in another ten to twenty years. "Just this once" is not a concept your skin understands; eventually, perhaps a decade later, you will see every minute of overexposure reflected in thickened, sagging, wrinkled skin, or possibly even in the growth of skin cancers.

Obviously, men with extremely fair skin have the least

amount of melanin present in the outer layer of the epidermis to begin with, and consequently they must be the most careful to limit their initial exposure. The darker your skin, the less risk you run, and black men, whose skin has already manufactured a great deal of protective pigmentation, can stay out longer than anyone else without damage. Still, as we mentioned earlier, even black skin can burn: at its most potent, melanin does not screen out *all* the sun's harmful rays. Moreover, the main function of melanin, as far as your body is concerned, is to provide protection for the delicate inner layers of the skin. The outermost layers, those we can see, will still become dehydrated, wrinkled, and leathery—tanned, in fact, like a hide—from chronic overexposure to the sun.

Guidelines for Tanning Safely

How, then, do you go about having your sun and maintaining healthy skin too? First, by working up to your tan very, very gradually, in order to allow the body to build up and deploy its melanin defenses. This means taking seriously the guidelines set out by the American Medical Association, and adhering to them, despite your impatience. They are as follows: if you are blond-haired, light-skinned, blue-eyed, restrict yourself to fifteen minutes in the sun the first day out, and increase the time by five minutes a day for the next three days. After that, you're on your own, advised only to be mindful of redness or tenderness. Dark-complected men simply augment the time by five minutes, beginning with twenty rather than fifteen. It is true that these guidelines were formulated for skin unprotected by sunscreens but, given the fact that even the best sunscreen provides only limited protection, they are still the rule of thumb for anyone who is seriously interested in maintaining the health of his skin.

Some other points to keep in mind: the sun's rays are the

most direct, and therefore, most dangerous, between 10 A.M. and, depending on Daylight Saving Time policies, either 2 or 3 P.M. Under these circumstances, it might make sense to get an early start, beginning your tanning at 9 or 9:30 in the morning, when you will be getting only about half as many ultraviolet rays—still plenty for the foundations of a tan; then seek shelter at around 10 o'clock. Of course, you are also aware that your skin is under greater pressure on the beach in, say, Puerto Rico or Miami than in Martha's Vineyard or San Francisco and, if you live in the northern hemisphere, in May, June, and July, than in January. (You may not be aware, however, that you run an even greater risk of burning in late May than in August, both because you are less likely to have an existing tan in May and because it is closer to the summer solstice on June 21.)

Remember, too, that altitude increases the intensity of the sun's rays, which is one of the things skiers must contend with, along with the fact that, even in the middle of winter, up to 85 percent of these rays will be reflected back at them from snow. Nonskiers should keep in mind that the same kind of reflection occurs with water and, to a lesser extent, sand; consequently you shouldn't think you're completely sheltered because you're sitting under a beach umbrella or a poolside awning. You will, by the way, also be vulnerable on hazy days. Although you may not feel their warmth directly, about 80 percent of those ultraviolet rays are being bounced down to you by tiny reflector drops of moisture in the atmosphere. Pollution, on the other hand, is, to some extent, impermeable to the sun's rays, which makes sunning on a city rooftop a bit safer for your skin, if not for your lungs or mental state.

Sunglasses are a must whenever you plan to be in the sun; not only do they protect your eyes from severe sun damage but they will, to some extent, keep those dehydrating rays off the already dry, extremely delicate skin tissue around the eye. Moreover, by reducing glare, they will reduce squinting, which can cause or exacerbate those tiny (or not so tiny) wrinkles around the eyes. You must also pay extra attention to your hair in the sun, especially if your scalp tends to be dry; a light woven cap will protect your hair and scalp from the sun's rays without trapping salt and perspiration which can also damage your hair.

These precautions, by the way, are not intended only for those who set out, singlemindedly, to acquire a tan. Men who, for whatever reason, spend a great deal of time outdoors, will suffer just as much from the sun's harmful rays as those who lie on the beach and bake. True, a seasoned outdoorsman will usually have a protective layer of tan to begin with, but he may also be less scrupulous about wearing screening lotions or the proper clothing to protect himself, under the mistaken notion that he has become invulnerable to the sun. As I said before, effective as the body's own defenses are, they cannot counteract for long years of abuse. Repeated overexposure not only alters the texture of the epidermis, or outer skin layer, but will eventually damage the supportive collagen. This, added to the dehydration that is already going on in the epidermis, increases the very real risk of skin cancers, an exorbitant price to pay for the dubious privilege of going unprotected in the sun.

Sunning Products

Use some kind of sun shield not only in the crucial early days of tanning, but whenever you plan to be in the sun for any length of time. You can make your own light, effective shield by mixing two parts peanut or wheat germ oil or mineral oil, two parts alcohol or vodka, and one part vinegar, placing these ingredients in a bottle and shaking well. If you like, you can also add a few drops of tincture of iodine to the mixture. Keep the bottle tightly closed and store it in a cool, dry place.

Once you're out in the sun, smooth the lotion over your skin, but don't rub it in; it must remain on the skin surface in order to shield you. Reapply often, as water and perspiration will wash it off.

The number of commercial sunscreens and other tanning products available is, in itself, mind-boggling. The selection is further complicated by the dizzying assortment of ingredients they contain and the promises (all too often misleading) they make. Should you decide to use a commercial product, however, look for a sunscreen containing PABA (para-aminobenzoic acid), the most effective screening ingredient on the market. Read the labels carefully until you find a product that suits your skin's special needs. First note the preparation's SPF, or Sun Protection Factor, the number that tells you how many times longer you can stay out in the sun when you use it than when you use nothing at all. This doesn't mean that you necessarily have to take advantage of those increments or that you should (with winter-white skin on a Caribbean beach) even trust them. But you can probably give yourself a little extra sun time, depending on the degree of protection your product affords.

Be especially wary when using products with a very low SPF, say 2 or 4, or those claiming to "promote deep tanning." This is at best an embellishment of the truth, since your skin tans at its own predetermined rate and the only point of any lotion is to help to keep it from burning in the process. Be careful, too, of products intended for people who "tan easily"; this simply means that these preparations offer very little sunscreen protection. On the other end of the spectrum are the sun blocks which, as the name implies, don't just screen but actually block the sun's rays. Sun blocks are useful for those with extremely sensitive skin, for anyone with a history of sun-related skin problems, and for specific, highly vulnerable or continually exposed areas, especially around the nose or eyes. A good, simple sun block is zinc oxide ointment, available at most drugstores. If the "clown" look that results from using this white ointment annoys you, at the very least use a product with a high (15+) SPF.

Whatever product you decide to use, be sure you first read the label carefully and gauge your exposure time accordingly. Use some sort of sunscreen whenever you plan to be in the sun and, especially in the early stages of your tan, remember to reapply the lotion thoroughly and often. Do not, however, expect PABA or any other screening ingredient to replace common sense. Nor, once out on the beach or the tennis courts, should you be tempted to tell yourself that you will go in at the first sign of a sunburn. The first sign will come too late to do your skin any good, since the extent of the burn will not begin to be visible for at least four hours after exposure, and its full effects may not make themselves felt for another twenty-four hours.

AFTER THE SUN

The first and most important thing to do after exposure is to cleanse your face, hair, and body thoroughly, to wash away salt, dirt, perspiration, and any chemicals left on your skin by pool water or commercial suntan products. Always bathe or shower with lukewarm, not hot, water. Cleanse your face with the lotion recommended for your skin type, and be sure to follow the cleansing with plenty of moisturizer, perhaps more than you think you need. Moisturize your entire body, being careful to use the recommended moisturizer for your face.

SUNBURN

What if, despite all your precautions or, at least, your best intentions, you burn anyway? To some extent, you will just have to let the burn run its course. Naturally, you should get out of the sun and stay out of it completely until the burn heals. Burns can range in severity from slight redness and soreness to considerable swelling and extremely painful blistering. If your burn is in the latter category, see a doctor immediately. A bad sunburn is a *burn;* it demands professional treatment or you may wind up with infections and even deep scarring. In the case of less serious sunburns, however, there are a number of preparations you can make yourself to ease the pain. Chamomile compresses, buttermilk compresses, Aloe Vera gel, or compresses made with boiled milk are all soothing to sunburned skin, while yogurt or sour cream applied directly will help reduce swelling. Or mix equal parts of milk, borax, and flour (a couple of tablespoonfuls of each should suffice), apply the mixture with compresses, and leave the compresses on for ten minutes. Rinse with milk.

PHOTOSENSITIVITY AND SUN-RELATED SKIN PROBLEMS

Sunburn, I'm afraid, is not the only immediate danger your skin has to face in the sun. You'll also have to watch out for photosensitivity, an umbrella word used to describe any number of abnormal reactions that develop as a result of your chemistry's being combined with substantial doses of sun. One common set of reactions has to do with prescription drugs, some of which markedly increase your skin's vulnerability to ultraviolet radiation. The trouble may show up either as a burn or a lesion, and can result in blistering and severe discomfort. Among the drugs that may make your skin more susceptible to sun damage are antibiotics, laxatives, diuretics, saccharine, tranquilizers, certain antihistamines, antifungal agents, and some diabetes, high blood pressure, and heart medications. If you're taking any prescription drug, it's best to check with your doctor before you venture out into the sun; he may suggest you avoid the sun completely for one, or even more, seasons.

Nor are drugs the only substances that can cause over-reaction to sun. Antibacterial deodorant soaps can also wreak havoc with your skin, especially in men over forty. And you should avoid using any product that contains fragrance when in the sun, since many of these can cause patches of irregular pigment or irritation in reaction to ultraviolet rays. Finally, some people find they have allergic reactions to ingredients contained in tanning preparations themselves. If you suspect you may be one of these people, your best bet is simply to stay away from commercial products, sticking instead to natural formulations such as the one I have described in this chapter.

Any man who has, or is prone to, couperose skin should avoid the sun completely. Excessive heat will only strain the fragile capillaries further, distending them to the breaking point and bringing them closer to the skin surface, where they are easily damaged. You should also go easy on midday plunges into a cold ocean or swimming pool, splashing your face with icy water to cool off, and other temperature extremes that accompany summer living.

ELEVEN

NUTRITION

ANYONE WHO wants good skin must begin by eating good food in the proper amounts. Your skin, after all, is a direct reflection of the state of your health; it is quick to show the effects of overeating or crash dieting, of excessive alcohol consumption, of foods loaded with toxins or lacking in nutrients, and it is markedly affected by even the subtlest vitamin and mineral deficiencies. Conversely, troubled skin is, in a sense, "telling" you something, serving as an early warning system for the body it sheathes, mirroring some internal distress. When your skin improves as a result of better nutrition, so does your health and your general sense of well-being.

Fortunately, Americans are becoming more and more aware of the relationship between diet and health and many people are beginning to try to incorporate sound nutritional principles into their everyday lives. But this is only the beginning, and for most of us, there is still plenty to learn. This is not, of course, a book about nutrition, so I won't take it on myself to spell out everything you need to know to eat properly to feel and look better; that would take an entire volume. (You can check the short list of recommended books at the end of this chapter for a fuller understanding of the foods we eat and their effect on our lives.) But I will give you some of the basic facts about nutrition, particularly as it applies to your skin.

PROTEIN

You probably know by now that it is essential to get enough protein in your diet, to keep saturated fats and cholesterol to a safe minimum, and to go easy on calories and carbohydrates if you want to keep your weight down. Complete proteins—those containing all the essential amino acids—are found in fish, poultry, meat, milk, yogurt, cheese, and eggs. Given the high rate of heart attacks and heart disease in America, however, it makes sense for a man to choose most of his proteins from the first two categories, since they are lower in saturated fats and cholesterol and, as a bonus, far lower in calories. In addition, you can get plenty of incomplete but high-quality protein from vegetables and whole grains, especially from beans, seeds and nuts, brown rice, wheat germ, and brewers' yeast, all of which are rich in crucial vitamins and minerals as well.

Why is so much emphasis placed on protein? In terms of our discussion, it is because your skin is largely made up of protein (as are your hair and nails); it is the protein structure in the dermis that gives your face its contours and elasticity, and a good supply of protein is necessary throughout your life to build and maintain skin cells and skin tissue.

FIBER

Another dietary factor that is crucial to your skin, and one we are only beginning to be aware of, is fiber. Fiber, or "roughage," consists of those parts of vegetable matter that can't easily be broken down by our digestive enzymes. Fiber forces waste products to move through your system and be excreted quickly and consistently; it ensures regular elimination and keeps your system from becoming sluggish, laden with toxins and harmful bacteria. In other words, fiber helps keep your system "clean" and unblocked, and it has precisely the same effect on your skin. Constipation and a body full of un-excreted toxins can cause acne, as well as a generally life-less-looking skin; and the job of taking care of your skin involves keeping it clean and unblocked from the inside as well as from the outside.

Unfortunately, few of us get enough fiber in our diets unless we make a conscious effort to do so. Modern milling and refining processes have taken the wheat bran out of our breads and cereals and it is precisely that bran which is the most concentrated—and the most traditional—source of fiber in an ordinary diet. Fortunately, however, there are now plenty of sources for whole-grain breads and cereals. These, by the way, are not only much better for you but, once you get used to them, you will find they taste better, too. You can also buy unprocessed miller's bran at most health food stores and sprinkle a teaspoonful or two on the foods you eat throughout the day for an equally beneficial effect. In addition, fresh fruits and vegetables provide roughage, especially when eaten raw, and a diet that includes plenty of these will also help keep your caloric intake down. Anyone interested in weight control, which is to say most of us, should make it a point to stick to a diet rich in high-fiber foods from each of these categories, since they are highly filling, relatively low in calories, extremely low in fats, and, by speeding the elimina-tion of waste, help you lose weight.

QUICK-WEIGHT-LOSS DIETS

Speaking of weight control, I can't warn you strongly enough against faddish quick-weight-loss diets. These operate by flushing water out of the body, so that while, in many cases, you will see a dramatic loss of pounds, you haven't really lost fat at all, and the weight will begin to creep back almost immediately. This in itself is not our problem, however; what *is* is the fact that the water lost is absolutely essential to the health of your skin. One of the goals of good skin care is to keep as much moisture as possible locked into the skin cells and to avoid dehydration. By causing extreme water loss, fad diets not only threaten, they absolutely ensure, disastrous dehydration of the skin cells, causing wrinkles, dry, dull skin, and premature aging. Moreover, any diet that causes you to shed pounds too quickly puts a terrible strain on your skin's support system, causing sags and pouches that are, in the end, as unattractive as, and far more permanent than, the extra pounds you could have lost safely through a more gradual, sensible, healthy diet.

Looking good and eating right do not demand miracles of self-discipline; they can be achieved by substituting foods rich in fiber and nutrients for "empty" calories and by altering your daily habits to bring the foods you eat into a healthy balance. Don't starve yourself; just start eating more wisely.

VITAMINS AND MINERALS

A word about the foods you eat: most of us assume that all foods contain vitamins and that simply by following the established nutritional charts we can get all the nutrients our bodies require. Unfortunately, this isn't quite true. Modern methods of processing and preserving often give us foods that look beautiful, but have very few natural nutrients left in them. Improper cooking, especially overcooking, makes matters worse, so that often, even with the best intentions, we end up eating foods that provide us with little more than bulk and weight. You can counteract this, to some extent, by buying only the freshest, highest quality foods, by shopping at reputable health food stores, and by cooking fragile foods such as vegetables for as little time as possible. Still, you won't always be able to be sure of what you are getting for your food dollars, and for this reason, it is probably a good idea to take vitamin and mineral supplements regularly. Familiarize yourself with the basic information on vitamins and minerals in this chapter, and you will be in a better position to judge just how many essential nutrients you can get from natural sources and which, if any, you will have to obtain from supplements. You will also know considerably more about how to choose the supplements you do take without spending money unnecessarily or loading your system with vitamins and minerals your body is in no position to use.

What gets most novice vitamin-watchers into trouble is balance. All vitamins and minerals work together and must always be in a correct balance. Taking an excess of one vitamin can create a deficiency in another; taking one without others needed for its absorption may render it useless. For instance, Vitamins B_1, B_2, B_6, and folic acid should always be taken in equal amounts. Taking a large corrective dose of Vitamin B_1, say 100 milligrams daily, can easily cause a corresponding deficiency of Vitamins B_2 or B_6. Since all the B-vitamins work together, taking large doses of any one of them increases your body's need for the others. Vitamin A and D supplements, of value to skin, eyes, and bones, will do you no good without additional Vitamin E, because only Vitamin E can prevent them from being oxidized within the body. Similarly, neither Vitamin A, D, or E can be absorbed unless unsaturated fatty acids are present at the same time. Calcium, phosphorus, and magnesium are three minerals that should always be taken in the correct balance. If you take too much phosphorus, calcium will be excreted in the form of a phosphate salt. This is a problem that affects nearly all of us, because the American diet is extremely rich in phosphorus, less so in calcium, and downright poor in magnesium. Without adequate magnesium to work with calcium, the calcium won't reach the bones, but will be deposited in the soft tissues. On top of all of this, you need Vitamin D in large amounts to further regulate calcium-phosphorus metabolism on a daily basis.

You can see that nutrition is no simple thing. I'm always delighted when my clients become interested in it, and I've never failed to see significant improvement in their health and looks when they begin to apply what they've learned to their own diets. Every skin type benefits, and there are cases in which diet is so inadequate to begin with that the skin condition can improve *only* through better nutrition. Now let's get down to the basics: vitamins and minerals. My recommendations apply only to teen-agers and adults, of course, not to growing children. (More detailed information on nutrition can be found in the books recommended at the end of the chapter.)

Vitamin A

Vitamin A is essential to the eyes and skin. People who work in offices under artificial light are particularly subject to Vitamin A deficiency, which causes lowered resistance to infection as well as night blindness. With regard to the skin, a Vitamin A deficiency can cause dryness, roughness, impetigo, boils, acne, blackheads, and dandruff, as well as excessively dry or brittle hair. Liver is probably the best source; carrot juice contains considerable Vitamin A, as well. Recommended dosage is between 10,000 and 25,000 units per day. Don't go much above 25,000 units without the supervision of a physician, since Vitamin A can be stored in the body and very large amounts can eventually become toxic.

Vitamin D

This vitamin is essential for metabolism of the minerals calcium and phosphorus, and hence, for building strong bones and teeth. And since calcium acts as a natural tranquilizer, a deficiency of Vitamin D may lead to the kind of nervous state that prompts so many people to use chemical tranquilizers. It used to be assumed that D was required only by children, but this has been proven false. We need it all our lives for healthy bones, especially as we grow older. The elderly do not shrink when they take enough Vitamin D and calcium. The best natural sources of Vitamin D are fish, fish oils, and Vitamin D-enriched milk. In direct sunlight Vitamin D can be produced directly on the skin, but only if there is a generous layer of skin oil on the surface (virtually impossible unless one bathes only about once a week) and provided you don't wash after exposure. As the late Dr. Erno Laszlo, the noted skin specialist, put it, "Since no one is going to go without washing, Vitamin D capsules have been invented!" Nutritionists recommend between 1,000 and 2,500 units daily. Be careful though; this is another case where large doses taken over a prolonged period can be toxic.

Vitamin E

Vitamin E is needed to keep Vitamins A and D from being oxidized, which is to say simply destroyed in the body. This is why experiments on the efficacy of Vitamin A in preventing blackheads and pimples have had such conflicting results. In many of them, Vitamin A was given without Vitamin E; consequently, the A didn't work. Vitamin E also prevents the destruction of the unsaturated fatty acids, Vitamin D, Vitamin K, and several hormones in the body. Dr. Hans Selye's experiments with premature aging showed that Vitamin E could also prevent wrinkles. It improves blood circulation and is essential for maintaining healthy muscles and skin cells. It can apparently prevent scars caused by acne conditions, as well as by cuts, burns, and other accidents. Clearly, Vitamin E is an important—even a crucial—nutrient in

many different ways, yet natural sources are rather limited.
The best are wheat germ and wheat germ oil, but since
Americans eat mostly breads and cereals made from refined
flour, which has been stripped of its wheat germ, it is a good
idea to take Vitamin E supplements regularly; the best are
undoubtedly based on d-alpha-tocopherol acetate or succin-
ate. A conservative dosage of between 100 and 200 IU (In-
ternational Units) should be enough from adolescence to
about age fifty. After that, as much as 600 or 800 IU may be
necessary to counteract diminished cellular function. And
the dosage should be increased during illness or following an
injury. One word of caution, however: a large, sudden influx
of Vitamin E tends to raise blood pressure temporarily, so
anyone already suffering from high blood pressure should
start with no more than 100 IU a day, and gradually increase
the amount to 200 or 300 IU over a period of months.

Vitamin F

Vitamin F is the name sometimes given to linoleic acid, an
essential polyunsaturated fatty acid. This acid is found in the
excellent cold pressed vegetable oils available in health food
stores, and in nuts and seeds; also in products made from
vegetable oils, such as salad dressings and mayonnaise. It is
called an *essential* fatty acid because, unlike other fats, it
cannot be synthesized from carbohydrates. No cell can exist
without such acids nor can the adrenal and sex hormones. It
is difficult to lose weight without such unsaturated fats, because they help to burn saturated body fat. And, of course,
unsaturated fats have been used for years as a way of reducing blood cholesterol.

Dry skin is frequently caused by a deficiency of Vitamin F;
without it, the glands will not produce the oil that dry skin so
desperately needs, and there is evidence that Vitamin F is
necessary for normal metabolism even of oily or acne type

skin. Recommended intake is around two tablespoonsful of vegetable oil daily, spread throughout the day. It can be obtained from cold pressed vegetable oils such as soy, walnut, safflower, sesame, peanut, corn, and sunflower. (Olive oil is not a good source of Vitamin F.) Obviously, eating moderate quantities of sesame seeds, sunflower seeds, peanuts, or walnuts will also supply Vitamin F. Wheat germ and wheat germ oil are also excellent sources. All of these foods can quickly grow rancid at room temperature, and must be refrigerated.

Vitamin K

Vitamin K is necessary for blood clotting, and can apparently help prevent fatal heart attacks. Dr. Carlton Fredericks cites evidence showing that Vitamin K supplements help protect the liver and blood of people who work with lead and those who must regularly take cinchophen or salicylates such as aspirin. You can get Vitamin K from eggs and green vegetables. This vitamin is also produced by healthy intestinal bacteria. Deficiencies are rare, and you shouldn't need supplements as long as you keep your intestines functioning properly by eating plenty of yogurt, milk, unsaturated fatty acids, and high fiber foods such as bran, and provided you are not taking oral antibiotics, which kill the beneficial intestinal bacteria.

Lecithin

Lecithin is of particular interest to us from the point of view of skin care because it helps maintain the healthy adipose tissue which gives the face its youthful contours. Beyond that, it is a constituent of every cell in the body, and is needed by every one of them. Made up of fat, unsaturated fatty acids, and the two important B-vitamins choline and inositol, it is a strong emulsifier with particular value in ensuring the absorption and utilization of all the fat-soluble vitamins. Heart disease caused by high cholesterol levels in the blood can be prevented by taking lecithin, since it reduces cholesterol level in the blood. Lecithin can be produced in the liver under ideal circumstances, when the diet contains sufficient amounts of Vitamins F and B_6, choline, inositol, and magnesium. Since there are very rarely sufficient amounts of these nutrients available, it makes sense to take a tablespoonful or two of lecithin daily, not least for its role in improving digestion and in helping the absorption of Vitamins A, D, and E. Granular lecithin is the most palatable form; liquid lecithin is usually the least expensive. Capsules contain so little as to be almost entirely useless. Lecithin is directly utilized in the burning of body fat, and there is evidence that it is absorbed by the body in such a way that it has no caloric value—so if you are on a diet you can ignore the sixty calories contained in a tablespoonful. Since it regulates fat metabolism, and the appearance of your skin depends on the activity of your oil glands, lecithin can probably benefit all types of skin, oily as well as dry.

The B Complex

There are several vitamins belonging to the B complex, all of them important to your skin. Those that have been completely identified, and which can be synthesized, are Vitamins B_1 (thiamine), B_2 (riboflavin), B_6 (pyridoxine), niacin (also called nicotinic acid. It is also available in a modified form called niacinamide, nicotinamide, or nicotinic acid amide; it is sometimes referred to as Vitamin B_3, and in Europe, as Vitamin PP), folic acid, pantothenic acid (calcium pantothenate), PABA (para-aminobenzoic acid), B_{12}, B_{15} (pangamate or calcium pangamate), biotin, choline, and inositol; twelve different factors in all. In addition, there are related nutrients called the antistress factors, which have not been completely identified, and which are available only from liver, kidney, soybeans, brewers' or torula yeast, wheat germ, and cooked green vegetables. The B-complex is absolutely essential for converting carbohydrates into energy. And given all the refined carbohydrates we eat today, all of which have been stripped of the B factors necessary to convert them into energy, it is especially important to take B-vitamin supplements. I cannot overemphasize that the B-vitamins all work together, and must all be present in the proper amounts if you plan to stay healthy. Before discussing the Bs separately, I'd like to point out that all of them have a direct influence on the skin, because of their ability to regulate oil gland secretions and control cell respiration.

Deficiency can cause oily and acne skin conditions, and burning, irritation, and wrinkles. The consumption of alcohol and all refined carbohydrates—especially sugar—causes Vitamin B-complex needs to skyrocket.

Vitamin B_1: This vitamin is necessary for normal growth. Deficiency causes numerous digestive disturbances, fatigue, and nervous irritability among other problems.

Vitamin B_2: B_2 is necessary for good vision, digestion, healthy blood, and in fighting the more serious skin diseases such as eczema and fungus infections. It is also important for the mucous membranes.

Vitamin B_6: Research is constantly uncovering new functions for B_6. Deficiency causes many skin disorders, headaches, intestinal cramps, gas, diarrhea, hemorrhoids, anemia, dandruff, hair loss, sore tongue, mental depression, water retention, insomnia, nervousness, fatigue, eczema, dyspepsia, arthritis, and a host of other nervous disorders. B_6 has also been found to regulate the critical balance of sodium and potassium in the body, which is why it has become so popular as a weight-loss aid. It is also essential for the natural production of lecithin.

Niacin and Niacinamide: Niacin deficiencies are not uncommon. Pellagra is the best known, but symptoms can range from depression, irritability, and even schizophrenia, to problems with the tongue, mouth, liver, and reproductive organs. A complete lack of niacin could even cause insanity. Although most of us get at least some niacin in our diets, it is probably not enough for optimum health. This vitamin comes in two forms—niacin and niacinamide; the latter is the one usually found in vitamin supplements, because it doesn't produce hot flushes, as ordinary niacin often does.

PABA: PABA is of great interest because of its ability to increase the skin's resistance to the sun. (This nutrient was discussed more fully in Chapter X on the sun.) Apparently it also has the ability to slow down aging. In the form of procaine, it is the principal agent in Dr. Anna Aslan's rejuvenation therapy. Innumerable reports have hailed its ability to return graying hair to its original color, although this requires large doses, and there is still some controversy over its effectiveness in this area. Success has also been reported in using PABA to treat eczema.

Pantothenic Acid: Pantothenic acid is considered to be the most important antistress vitamin, in part because it helps prevent exhaustion of the adrenal glands. A lack of pantothenic acid prevents the adrenal glands from producing the cortisone that is necessary to combat stress, and may also cause low blood sugar (or hypoglycemia, the no-energy disease), susceptibility to allergies and infections, graying hair, and any number of skin problems, including granulation of the sensitive eyelid tissue.

Folic Acid: This is one of the most important B factors, and one least often supplied in adequate amounts, largely because it is easily destroyed in food, and because the FDA limits its sale in this country to an extremely small quantity. A recent government survey on nutrition found that many Americans suffer from a deficiency of folic acid, so perhaps now the FDA will allow us to obtain larger quantities of this vital nutrient. Since folic acid is needed for many of the same reasons as other members of the B complex, folic acid deficiency leads to pernicious anemia, low digestive acid levels, and liver malfunction. Its lack can also be a factor in baldness.

Biotin: Since it is usually assumed that adequate biotin is manufactured by the intestines, only small-dose tablets are available. This is fine as long as intestinal bacteria are functioning properly, which is not always the case, especially when antibiotics are taken. As with folic acid, very large doses are freely available in Europe, and studies showing the efficacy of external biotin treatments in treating male baldness suggest that we may not be getting as much of this vitamin as we should. Biotin also helps prevent eczema, lung infections, dry, peeling skin, muscular pain and fatigue, and inadequate growth (it is a potent cell stimulant). It is found in liver and in brewers' yeast, the best source for all the B vitamins.

Vitamin B_{12}: This vitamin has been used for years as a quick energy booster, yet no one knows why it has such dramatic effects. Unless you are a strict vegetarian, you probably don't have to worry about deficiencies of this vitamin, since the body's requirements are relatively small and easily obtainable from natural sources.

Choline and Inositol: The body requires substantial amounts of both these vitamins, yet the average diet supplies very little. Refining largely eliminates them from foods, and enriching doesn't put them back. Nutritionists often recommend 500 to 3,000 milligrams of each per day. Lecithin is our richest source; a tablespoonful of granular lecithin contains 250 milligrams of each, while a tablespoonful of the less palatable liquid variety contains 375 milligrams. Interestingly enough, the body requires large amounts of choline and inositol to produce its own lecithin. Choline is necessary for healthy functioning of the liver, kidneys, nerves, and muscles, and for the synthesis of nucleic acids in the cells. Choline supplements have also relieved high blood pressure. Inositol is important for liver function and also for vision. Deficiency can cause eczema and other skin disorders. Inositol has recently attracted attention as an effective substitute for chemical tranquilizers, and has been used, with varying degrees of success, in treating baldness.

B Complex Formula: Your body requires that the B vitamins be supplied in a very specific ratio, a fact which is often ignored by the makers of vitamin supplements. The late Adelle Davis devised an excellent formula for B-complex tablets that very few nuritionists would quarrel with. It is quite conservative compared to the megadoses some nutritionists are now recommending, but it respects the body's needs and does not oversupply when there is no clear necessity. The formula Davis recommended contains the following: 5 milligrams each of folic acid, B_1, B_2, and B_6; 30 milligrams of pantothenic acid, niacinamide, and PABA; 1,000 milligrams each of choline and inositol; 15 micrograms of B_{12}, and 25 micrograms of biotin. This formula has become very popular with knowledgeable vitamin buyers; it is availble at all health food stores and from a number of manufacturers, sometimes with slight modifications. And again, healthy intestines will manufacture the right proportions of the B complex, provided you stick to an extremely wholesome diet that is especially rich in yogurt and fiber, whole grains, liver, wheat germ, and brewers' yeast.

Vitamin C

Millions of Americans have been taking large, even massive doses of Vitamin C on a regular basis ever since Dr. Linus Pauling's highly publicized findings that C could prevent and cure the common cold. Most people are still unaware, however, of its enormous effect on the skin. Collagen cannot be formed without adequate Vitamin C. Since the sagging that accompanies age is caused by degeneration of the dermis, it seems logical that this could be delayed or avoided by ensuring consistent and adequate C intake all your life. Moreover, Vitamin C and the C related factors—bioflavinoids, hesperidin, and rutin—regulate the strength and permeability of the capillary walls, thus preventing broken capillaries. Vitamin C is of value in every disease caused by virus or bacteria. It can detoxify harmful side effects of virtually every drug (even aspirin), and of many metals. It can also apparently largely detoxify cigarette smoke. It has been estimated that 25 mg. of Vitamin C are used up with every cigarette. It is also one of the antistress vitamins. You can always tell you have a C deficiency if you bruise easily; Vitamin C largely prevents bruises, and promotes extremely rapid healing of them. Vitamin C has been reported to cure allergies, and can apparently treat such skin diseases as poison ivy and poison oak. C, of course, was originally discovered when citrus fruits were found to cure scurvy. And Dr. Walter Eddy of Columbia University showed that many of the symptoms of old age are identical to those of scurvy, and these include wrinkles and loss of elasticity in the dermis. However, C is just as important to the teen-ager suffering from acne, because it helps prevent acne scarring in the dermal layer. By the same token, it should be taken whenever the skin is more seriously injured: in cases of wounds, burns, and before and after surgery. Strawberries, guavas, and mangoes are also rich in C. Cabbage, especially in the form of sauerkraut, and green vegetables are good sources as long as the vegetables are cooked quickly in little water, and the cooking water is served along with the vegetable.

Most nutritionists would recommend supplementing your diet with daily Vitamin C tablets. Enthusiasts recommend 500 to 2,500 milligrams daily, but this seems a little high to me. Yet there is much evidence to show that 100 milligrams a day is not enough. Certainly large doses should be taken when you are ill or under stress, as in the antistress formula I'll discuss later on in this chapter. Normally, however, I don't think you should take more than 200 or 300 milligrams per day, unless, of course, you smoke. It is wise to remember that fads exist in science and medicine as anywhere else.

It is possible that our Vitamin C needs could be greatly reduced by taking large quantities of the C-related factors, the bioflavinoids, rutin, and hesperidin, also known as Vitamin P. In many cases where Vitamin C was not doing as much as it should, adding Vitamin P has dramatically increased its effectiveness. Vitamin P also strengthens tiny capillaries (Vitamin C has more effect on the larger blood vessels) and is therefore particularly important to anyone with a tendency toward couperose skin. Good sources for Vitamin P are—assuming they are fresh and of high quality—apricots, blackberries, black currants, cabbage, cherries, grapes, grapefruit, lemons, oranges, plums, prunes, and rose hips. Unstrained citrus juice is much higher in bioflavinoids than strained citrus juice, and all the white filaments and pulp of citrus fruits are exceptionally rich sources; thus it makes more sense to eat your citrus whole than juiced. Since natural sources often contain a hundred times as much Vitamin P as Vitamin C, the body's requirements for P are probably far greater. So, when buying Vitamin C tablets, be sure that they contain at least the same quantity of bioflavinoids as of C, and at least one tenth that amount of rutin, and preferably of hesperidin as well.

Calcium

This mineral is essential for the health of bones, teeth, and the neuromuscular system. It is also responsible, along with Vitamin C, for building the collagen, or elastic tissue, that supports our skin. Deficiency can cause nervousness, irritability, and insomnia. Many use calcium as a tranquilizer: one or two grams taken before bedtime with magnesium will promote restful sleep without the hangovers and serious side effects of drugs. Adequate Vitamin D, Vitamin E, and magnesium must be present in the diet in order for calcium to be utilized properly by the body. And if there is too much phosphorus in the diet (and there nearly always is in the average American diet), calcium will be excreted.

In addition to its action in building the protein of the dermis, calcium may have an effect on the outer skin layer—the epidermis—since it is a constituent of the skin's Natural Moisturizing Factor, or NMF. The body's supply of NMF dwindles as we grow older, leading to aging of the skin through dehydration. It is possible that one of the contributory factors in reduced NMF production is a lack of calcium in the diet, an insufficient supply of Vitamins D and E and magnesium necessary for its utilization, or an overabundance of phosphorus that nullifies calcium intake.

The US RDA for calcium is 1 gram or 1,000 milligrams daily, which should be adequate for most people. Milk is the most frequently used dietary source. Calcium is also found in oranges, green leafy vegetables, wheat germ, cheese, soybeans, sesame seeds, and yogurt. Amino acid chelated calcium is probably the best supplemental form to take, preferably combined with magnesium in a 2:1 ratio.

By the way, the unsightly calcium deposits that can be seen in aging skin are not caused by too much calcium, but rather from poorly utilized calcium. Even if there is no calcium in the diet at all, deposits can occur when this nutrient is withdrawn from the bones and is not metabolized correctly. Adequate Vitamin E and magnesium will prevent and eliminate these deposits.

Phosphorus

Like calcium, phosphorus is required for bones, teeth, and the neuromuscular system. It is also important for normal brain development. Of all nutrients, it is the one most likely to be supplied in abundance. In fact, that's where the problem lies. Virtually every food except pure fat and pure sugar contains phosphorus. And whenever phosphorus is oversupplied, calcium is excreted, creating serious health problems. Phosphorus must combine with calcium to be utilized by the bones. When calcium is not present in the body, but phosphorus is, the body will take the calcium it needs from the bones, making them brittle and leading to severe tooth decay.

Magnesium

This mineral, extremely undersupplied in our diet, is important in all calcium functions, since calcium cannot work without it. It is also known for its tranquilizing effect, and for promoting good elimination. Because modern agricultural methods prevent plants from absorbing magnesium from the soil, you should take some kind of supplement. Remember that the ideal balance between calcium and magnesium is two parts calcium to one part magnesium. The minimum daily requirement for magnesium is 300 millligrams daily, and multi-amino-acid chelated mineral tablets supplying this amount as well as 600 milligrams of calcium and other minerals are readily available.

Zinc

Check your fingernails. If you can see white spots on them, chances are you have a zinc deficiency. Zinc is an important mineral for a number of reasons, not least of which is its reported usefulness in controlling and eliminating acne. It stimulates and hastens the healing of all skin diseases, scars, burns, and surgical incisions and it is essential to growth and sexual development. Deficiencies are common, causing susceptibility to infection, infertility, and, possibly, acne. Also important for men is the fact that zinc can prevent or cure enlarged prostate gland conditions.

The US RDA is 15 milligrams daily, although as much as 30 milligrams would probably be a better level. Natural sources include liver and wheat germ.

Iron

Iron is essential to the formation of hemoglobin, the carrier of oxygen in the red blood cells. Serious fatigue can result from even a borderline deficiency. It used to be assumed that grown men in this country had little need of supplemental iron, but recent government surveys show that millions of American men suffer from iron deficiency. Liver is the only extremely rich natural source, and everyone suffering from any kind of anemia can benefit from its blood-building properties, some of which are due to as yet unknown factors. Those of us who do not eat liver (or a grain particularly rich in iron, such as millet and wheat germ) daily will need iron supplements. Daily doses of 15 to 20 milligrams are considered to be an average requirement, and you shouldn't take more without the advice of your physician. Certain types of iron supplements, particularly ferrous sulfate and ferrous chloride, can apparently destroy Vitamin E, but the form of iron used in top-quality multiple supplements is usually safe.

Sodium and Potassium

These minerals regulate the fluids in your body. Sodium is supplied by table salt (sodium chloride), and by thousands of processed foods and food additives. Potassium is found in fruit, vegetables, grains, and beans.

Too much sodium creates a potassium deficiency, and vice versa. Excessive sodium causes high blood pressure and water retention or edema; too much potassium creates low blood pressure and dehydration of the cells. The basis of most quick-weight-loss diets is an abundance of high-potassium foods, or other foods that cause sodium to be lost. These diets cause excretion of the sodium and water found naturally in every cell of your body. While they can allow you to lose up to five pounds in a very short time, the weight will come back almost immediately. What's worse, quick-weight-loss diets can do irreversible damage to your skin. As the deeper skin cells become dehydrated, tone is lost, and rapid aging of the skin results.

Our biggest problem, however, is inadequate potassium. According to recent government surveys, this may be the most serious health problem in our country. We don't, on the whole, eat as much of the potassium-rich foods as we should, and processed foods (this includes canned and frozen vege-tables) almost invariably have a great deal of unnecessary sodium added. Besides the danger of hypertension, which can lead to stroke (for the relationship between hypertension and couperose skin, see Chapter VI), a low potassium level can cause low blood sugar, hypoglycemia, with its attendant fatigue, loss of energy, and other symptoms.

The obvious solution is to cut your intake of salt and salty foods to the absolute minimum, especially in winter, when there is no danger of heat stroke, and to eat as many fresh fruits and vegetables as possible, perhaps two or three servings of vegetables at every meal. Vegetables should be cooked in as little water as possible. Hypertension can largely be avoided by reducing salt intake and emphasizing foods rich in potassium. You can never start too soon; research has shown that babies given highly salted prepared foods will later have a predisposition to hypertension. And excessive sodium will tax the kidneys to an extent which will eventually encourage serious kidney disease. Have your blood pressure checked. If it is too high, you're probably getting too much salt and too little potassium.

Iodine

Iodine is essential to the thyroid gland, which regulates your body functions. An underactive thyroid can make you fat, cause dry skin, and make hair fall out, among other things. People with acne, however, are advised to avoid iodine. I am not sure that this is a good idea, since iodine is such an important nutrient. If you have acne, your best bet is probably to experiment: try making your diet adequate in every other respect for at least a month, then add an iodine supplement for a week and see if it causes breakouts. You cannot live without iodine indefinitely, so if you do break out, you will have to experiment every two months or so, until you can take iodine safely. One thing that may help is making sure you take plenty of Vitamin E, which dramatically increases your body's ability to absorb iodine. Iodine is found in iodized salt, seafood, kelp, sea salt, and spinach.

Chromium

Although this mineral is needed in only tiny amounts, deficiencies are widespread, since modern agricultural and refining methods have almost eliminated it from our diet. It helps the body utilize sugar normally, and those who eat a lot of sugar have a far higher requirement for it. Chromium is now included in nearly all the good amino-acid-chelated multimineral supplements. Recommended intake is 0.25 milligrams (250 micrograms) to 3 milligrams daily.

Manganese

Manganese is one of the nutrients most important to tissue respiration and, therefore, to healthy skin. It is also necessary for proper functioning of the brain, glands, and reproductive organs, for lowering cholesterol, for muscle coordination, bone formation, sugar and fat metabolism, and normal growth, as well as for utilization of Vitamins B_1 and E. Wheat germ is an extremely rich source.

Selenium

Although this mineral is becoming popular, little is known about it except that it is an antioxidant and shares many other qualities with Vitamin E. The best sources are brewers' yeast and liver. Like so many other minerals, selenium has been refined and processed out of most foods. Supplements are available in health food stores, usually combined with Vitamin E. Now that selenium is being used in research on heart disease, this nutrient will probably begin to receive more public attention. It may also have an effect on dandruff, oily skin, and acne, since selenium salts are widely used in dandruff shampoos.

Recommended Reading

Davis, Adelle, *Let's Get Well,* New York; New American Library/Signet, 1972
Dufty, William, *Sugar Blues,* New York; Warner Books, 1976
Kushi, Michio, *Natural Healing Through Macrobiotics,* New York; Japan Publications, 1977

Lappé, Francis Moore, *Diet For A Small Planet,* revised edition, New York; Ballantine Books, 1975

Null, Gary, *Protein for Vegetarians,* revised edition, New York; Jove Publications, 1975

Null, Gary and Steven, *The New Vegetarians,* New York; Dell Publishing, 1973

Williams, Roger J., *Nutrition Against Disease,* New York; Bantam Books, 1973

TWELVE

THE WAY WE LIVE

I HAVE NEVER cared for the word lifestyle. It has always struck me as superficial, empty, a way of designating something less than true *personal* style. But even I must admit that there are times when the term is indispensable. And now, as I near the end of this book on how to take good and proper care of your skin, is one of those times. For no other word sums up so succinctly the pressures and pleasures peculiar to life in this last quarter of the twentieth century—pressures and pleasures that have everything to do with how you look and feel.

Lifestyle is, I think, the sum of one's habits, outlooks, and susceptibilities, the way each of us approaches the myriad options available to him. I won't attempt to advise you on most of them, but a few—those concerning the care of your skin—are extremely important.

DRINKING AND SMOKING

Let's start with drinking, smoking, and drug-taking. Alcoholic beverages raise your breathing rate, which in turn causes your skin temperature to drop, which in turn enlarges your pores. The alcohol in liquor, wine, and beer also causes vasodilation, or expansion of the blood vessels. Drink enough such beverages over a prolonged period of time and the blood vessels will become permanently enlarged. Nor does the trouble end there: enlarged pores and dilated blood vessels, apart from being unsightly themselves, stretch the skin, making it sag and wrinkle. If you have any doubts about the effects of an overfondness for alcohol, take a look at the complexion of anyone you happen to know who drinks more than is good for him. Chances are, you'll then want to control your intake of alcohol.

Smoking is no less damaging to the skin. One California doctor, after studying well over a thousand smokers and nonsmokers, concluded that wrinkling of the skin of the face is yet another of the side effects (of which the list is growing constantly) of smoking. His report also pointed out that cigarette smokers have complexions which tend toward the yellow-gray, as opposed to the pink or the ruddy, in color. Finally, the simple act of puffing on a cigarette distorts the mouth hundreds of thousands of times over the course of a lifetime of smoking. Is it any wonder that smokers' mouths tend to be surrounded by fine lines?

Now, you are probably wondering if I am suggesting that you give up drinking and smoking altogether. Well, I'd never try to dissuade you from giving them up—smoking, especially, which has, after all, been linked to cancer and which doesn't even have the helpful capacity to reduce stress and worry, as one or two cocktails in the evening have been shown to do. But I would urge you to monitor your consumption of both alcohol and tobacco, to note how much of both you consume in the next few weeks. I've seldom met a man who didn't have a sense of how much was too much, even if he chose to ignore it. If *your* sense of moderation tells you that you're overstepping the bounds of good health, please pay attention to that sense. Skin is my primary concern, and I can assure you that if you're drinking and smoking to excess, irremedial changes in skin tone and color are only one of the afflictions being visited upon your body.

DRUGS

A word or two about drugs, especially sleeping pills. Obviously, dependence on them is dangerous. It's common knowledge that drug-induced sleep is different from normal sleep, and that anyone who takes medication to combat insomnia is harnessing himself to a potential addiction. For one thing, sleeping pills (including barbiturates and hypnotics) change the composition of the blood, and with it, of the skin. They also render tissues less elastic, which results in premature wrinkling. Dehydration, rashes, and appetite loss are other side effects of the regular taking of sleeping pills. I don't have to tell you at this point that they are natural enemies of a healthy, normal, young-looking complexion. If you're plagued by insomnia, see a doctor, visit a sleep clinic, or read a good book on the subject. They'll all tell you, in no uncertain terms, that pills are no better than a last resort, and they'll fill you in on alternative methods (including natural tranquilizers, such as Vitamin D, calcium, and magnesium) of achieving dependable, regular, trouble-free sleep.

SLEEP AND RELAXATION

While I'm on the subject of sleep, let me state what may be the obvious, but what, in our high-pressure, high-speed society, bears constant restating: sleep is one of the most important factors in maintaining a healthy body and a healthy complexion. My recommendation is that you should try to sleep between seven and eight hours a night, and that, maybe once a week, you get as much as nine or ten hours. While sleep needs do vary greatly (and do decrease with age), it's imperative that you not short-change yourself on this score. When it comes to preventing wrinkles, shadows and puffiness around the eyes, and maintaining good skin texture, there's nothing as effective as a good night's sleep. Closely related to ample sleep is the necessity for relaxation. This means that sometimes, even in the middle of the day or during the hours after you get home from work but before you begin your evening, you must force yourself to relax a bit. Easier said than done? Of course. But reducing tension before it's built to a crescendo is a good way to avoid lines of weariness and stress on the face—and all the other bodily ills that unrelieved, day-in-day-out anxiety can cause. A short nap, as short as fifteen minutes, will help. So will sitting with your head back and your feet elevated.

There are other ways of relaxing that you may not know about, and because they're so beneficial to the skin, I want to tell you about them. One way is to give yourself a facial, like the one I outline in Chapter VIII. If you don't have time for the full-scale facial (which, you may recall, can easily take half an hour), a ten-minute mask will prove a good substitute. Of course you'll lie down for this, and afterwards you'll feel refreshed *and* relaxed. The second way to relax is to treat yourself to a warm and moisturized bath, the kind I describe in Chapter IX.

Exercises for Relaxation

Facial exercises are the third way to relax. When you feel tension building in your forehead, when your eyes are strained and tired, when stress seems concentrated in any area of your face, exercises can go far toward relieving the tightness, the weariness. And while I don't believe that facial exercises can strengthen muscle weakness that comes from the aging process, or alter the natural contours of your face, they will make you look better as well as feel better. They do this by stimulating blood circulation in the face and neck, by toning both muscles and tissues. Tone, it goes without say-

ing, is important to anyone interested in projecting his vitality, and is the natural enemy of sagging, falling, "fleshy"
skin.

Before I give you specific exercises for all the regions of
your face—forehead, eyes, mouth, chin, and neck—let me suggest that you practice each exercise you choose to do in front
of the mirror until you do all the movements easily and naturally. As with any exercise, form is important; it means you'll
get the most out of the exercise. And having the correct form
actually serves to make the exercise *easier.* Soon you won't
need the mirror at all, which means you can do the exercises
at your desk or in the back seat of a taxicab. But, please, exercise no more than five or ten minutes a day; more than that
and you risk stretching the skin too much. Your attitude
should be one of concentration, but not overintensity.

For the forehead: Raise your eyebrows as high as you
can, then lower them very, very quickly. Repeat eight times.

For the eyes: Turn your eyes all the way to the right,
then to the left. Roll your eyes all the way up, then down.
Then blink, hard. A more extreme form of this exercise calls
for standing about six feet away from a wall (preferably
painted a solid color) so that you can see the entire wall.
Don't move your head, but do move your eyes, beginning at
the wall's upper righthand corner, in a clockwise direction,
down to the floor, advancing to the lower left corner, finally
raising the eyes to the upper left corner. Repeat ten times,
starting in the upper right corner and proceeding clockwise
five times, then in the upper left corner and proceeding
counterclockwise the other five. Then look up to the ceiling
and, very suddenly, look down to the floor; again, repeat ten
times. Finally look from the right half of the wall to the left
and back again, ten times. This relaxes the eyes and the
wrinkles that are one of the features of weary eyes.

For the mouth: Inhale quite deeply and hold the air in your mouth to a ten count, then release suddenly. Move your tongue in circles around the inside of your mouth. Finally, yawn in an exaggerated manner, opening your mouth as wide as possible.

For the chin: Move your lower jaw back and forth, and from side to side, ten times. Turn your head all the way to the right, then all the way to the left, ten times. Stretch your head backward, as far as it will comfortably go; then place your lower lip over the upper one and slowly open and close your mouth; ten times. This is especialy good for discouraging a double chin, but will also relax the entire head/neck area.

For the neck: Make a complete circle with your neck, rotating it twenty times in a clockwise direction, and twenty times in a counterclockwise one. Inhale deeply, bending the neck backward; then exhale, bending the neck forward.

REGULAR EXERCISE

While I'm on the subject of these simple and highly specific exercises for face and neck, let me stress what many, many experts in a variety of fields have spent much of the Seventies stating: regular exercise of an appropriate and fairly strenuous nature is vital to bodily health and to a feeling of personal well-being. From my own point of view as a skin-care specialist, exercise keeps the blood moving and allows the skin to breathe, and is most effective when undertaken in fresh air. Whenever possible, when exercising at home or in the gym, open the window wide. If it's cold, just dress accordingly. You'll immeasurably increase the benefits to be derived from the exercise.

I do have a very definite attitude toward any exercise program, and that is that it should be well rounded. There seems to be a tendency these days, among young men particularly, to tone, firm, and build muscle without paying simultaneous attention to the cardiovascular aspects of body fitness. Maintaining the health and efficiency of the circulatory system, the heart and blood vessels, and the lungs is immensely important. Jogging is probably the single most popular cardiovascular exercise, but bicycling, swimming, and even rope-skipping fulfill the same basic function: they make your heart beat faster, your breathing become deeper, and your blood vessels expand and open up to carry oxygen and blood to the working muscles of the body. A regular program of such exercise improves your body's ability to consume, transport, and utilize oxygen. For that reason, aerobic (from the Greek word for air) is another adjective often applied to such activities. More specifically, aerobic exercise steadily supplies sufficient oxygen to the exercising muscles for the duration of the exercise. Any activity that is rhythmic, repetitive, and dynamic and that can be continued for two or more minutes, without huffing and puffing afterwards, is probably aerobic and, with any luck, will confer cardiovascular benefits.

Physical fitness is widely held to have five critical—and readily distinguished—components: body composition (specifically, a proper proportion of fat to total body weight), flexibility, muscular strength, muscular endurance, and cardiovascular endurance. Why do I emphasize the last so much? In part because it seems to me to be the factor that most influences longevity and overall health, at least in our society, where there is so much encouragement *not* to walk, *not* to climb stairs, *not* to breathe deeply. But I'm also very definitely reacting to something I've observed in my many years of caring for the skin of men and women of all ages and all degrees of physical vitality. And that is simply this: skin is never healthy, never glowing, never youthful where circulation of the blood—that fluid charged with the conveying and distributing of oxygen and nutrients to all parts of the body—is in anything but first-rate condition. I can't help but think that what I see so clearly and so consistently with regard to the skin must be equally valid in regard to all the organs, muscles, and nerves that are hidden beneath it. And that is why I urge you not only to increase your flexibility and build your muscles, but to pay especially close attention to cardiovascular endurance.

I won't attempt to advise you on the correct exercise program for you, but you'll want to make sure that it includes all five of the physical fitness components I mention above. Many excellent books have been written about exercise and exercise programs. One, *Rating the Exercises*, by Charles T. Kuntzleman and the editors of *Consumer Guide* (William Morrow and Co., $10.95), gives pros and cons of everything from yoga to calisthenics, jogging to vibrator belts (these are useless, by the way). It also includes a chapter on finding a good health club. I suggest that, if you're beginning a fitness regimen in earnest, you take a look at this guide. I suggest, too, that you see your physician before your first workout, certainly if you're over the age of thirty.

Finally, whenever you jog, cycle, play tennis, or undertake any exercise outdoors, be sure to apply sunscreen and/or moisturizer, the former to combat the sun's ultraviolet rays, the latter the effects of cold and wind. By now, you know the reasons why. But it's easy to forget the lotion or cream in the excitement of heading for the track or court. And it's imperative that you *not* forget!

PROBLEMS OF INDOOR LIVING

So much of twentieth-century life is lived indoors, where artificial lighting and ventilation and climate control hold sway.

While I've had considerable opportunity to address myself to the special problems of the outdoorsman in the chapter on sun, its benefits and its curses, I've not had much chance to discuss the special problems of the "indoorsman"—the office worker, the apartment dweller.

Essentially, the problems are the by-now familiar ones of heat and air conditioning. Let me remind you of what I've already had to say on this subject: it is of the utmost importance that you keep your skin—if it is dry or even normal—moisturized in such an environment. Offices and apartments can, in the dead of winter or the heat of summer, be hard on the skin, as brutal as a ski slope in terms of sheer extremes of climate. Since you're a man, and since you probably don't have even the dubious protection that makeup affords, you must keep your skin moisturized. A humidifier in your bedroom or executive suite is, as I've suggested, a useful adjunct. But your after-shave moisturizer is still your best single protection.

Fluorescent lighting is another common aspect of office life that threatens a healthy skin. Some doctors maintain, for instance, that it can cause brown spots on the skin of face and hands by triggering a melanin reaction not dissimilar to the one that occurs on the beach in the middle of July. I don't know about that, but I do know that fluorescent lights can make the eyes unnaturally tired by the end of the working day, and I refer you to the formulary for a preparation that will soothe eyes that sting, ache, or merely feel weary. As for the sedentary way of life that an indoor life imposes on one, let me mention again the importance for all men and women, no matter what their age, to devise a suitable exercise program and stick to it.

But however you live, indoors or outdoors, boldly or cautiously, with an eye toward change or a deep respect for tradition, the information I've given in this chapter only supports the basic beliefs and assumptions that are the theme of this book. They are the same beliefs and assumptions that I have lived by during my twenty-five years as a chemist and skin-care specialist.

A FINAL MESSAGE

By "beliefs and assumptions" I don't mean simply things like soap is harmful to the complexion, or that Vitamin E can have a variety of beneficial effects on the skin when applied topically, or that too much sun—whether in the course of a day or in the course of a lifetime—is bad for you. All of those are useful working principles, of course, and as such, they matter to me deeply.

But I'm getting at something much more basic here, and it's the message that I am most interested in leaving with you. It's this: when you set out to take care of your skin—that wonderful membrane, so delicate yet so resolute—you needn't embrace doctrines, procedures, or preparations that don't make absolute sense to you. Yes, you must be open-minded. But there's no reason to subscribe to complicated regimens or to spend hundreds of dollars on exclusively formulated, elaborately packaged, department-store purveyed preparations. Far easier, far better, and far cheaper to follow the simplest of regimens, using preparations that you've made yourself, according to the instructions I've given you throughout the book and in the formulary. By making these preparations, combining these ingredients, feeling them on your fingertips, you come to understand them. You begin to develop and trust your own good instincts, based on personal experience.

There's no reason why skin care shouldn't be scientific, commonsensical, and natural all at the same time. And there's every reason why it should. Nor is there any defense for your being at the mercy of an outside force—be it cosmetics house or facialist—who asks you to do things you don't fully understand, that don't feel right. You are more than capable of taking charge of this important aspect of your body, your health, and your image. I know, because I have seen other men do so—men whose skin announces, more effectively than any expensive wristwatch, impressive professional title, or engraved business card ever could, the vitality, self-reliance, and clarity of vision they bring to every job they undertake.

FORMULARY

THROUGHOUT this book, I have been promising you the opportunity to make your own products—from cleansing lotions and the other basics in daily skin care to more specialized products like acne disincrustation compresses and warm wax masks. As I'm sure I've already made very clear, these products will be *natural* products, made from natural ingredients, all of which you can purchase at the supermarket, the drugstore, or the health foods store—and sometimes at all three.

Why my penchant for the all-natural? Let me say it again. The skin absorbs and accepts natural substances most easily. They are less likely to cause allergic reactions. Natural oils not only penetrate the skin, they *nourish* it—something mineral oil, baby oil, and petroleum jelly are incapable of doing. On the practical side, natural ingredients are readily available; they are also inexpensive. Because you are making your own products at home, they are of assured freshness, and do not need to be provided with a shelf-life via chemical preservatives. Finally, natural products are simple to prepare, fun to use, and, perhaps most important psychologically, they put you in touch with the essence of your own individualized skin-care regimen.

I'll provide formulations for specific products and specific skin types, of course, but first let me list the utensils you'll most likely need, and generalize a bit on ingredient families, as well as on such topics as storage.

UTENSILS AND INGREDIENTS

The utensils you'll require include a mixer—either electric or hand-held—and a blender; you'll use the latter to make juices from vegetables and fruits, and to blend and emulsify liquids. In addition you'll need saucepans (glass or enameled), including two that fit together as a double boiler. Avoid aluminum, tin, or tin-lined copper pots, which can change the composition of some of your ingredients. A few eyedroppers to measure truly small quantities of liquids; a set of measuring spoons; a four-cup measuring cup (marked in ounces); wooden or Plexiglas stirring spoons; funnels for decanting lotions; strainers; and a section of cheesecloth will complete your collection of essential utensils.

The ingredients that you'll be using are most often from the vegetable kingdom, and include fruits (grapefruits, lemons, oranges, apricots, strawberries); vegetables (cucumbers, carrots, tomatoes); herbs (dill, chamomile); seeds, grains, flours, and cereals and starches. Plants are often used specifically for their vitamin value, especially in nourishing creams and lotions. For instance, Vitamin A, found in fresh carrots, when added to a nourishing cream, keeps skin smooth and supple. Vitamin E, so abundant in vegetable oils, many dairy products, and egg yolk, helps combat wrinkling. Do make sure that the fruits and vegetables you use are absolutely fresh; the fresher they are, the more potent the vitamins they contain.

Some classes of ingredients require some comment. The first is alcohol, called for in small amounts in many of the formulas that follow. Essentially, I believe that you should use either ethanol or domestic vodka (isopropyl rubbing alcohol is almost always made synthetically, while foreign vodkas are very often flavored or scented.) Ethanol, available in this country primarily by prescription, is obviously stronger than the vodka; it also has a strong aroma of its own. If you are interested in gentleness *and* odorlessness, try the vodka which, while more expensive, will be used in such small quantities that it shouldn't amount to more than a few cents extra per month. Finally, and this is important, feel free to experiment with the alcoholic content of your preparations, within certain limits. If your prescribed formula is too strong for your skin type (if it dries, stings, or reddens your skin unduly), add a little water, which has been boiled, to dilute the strength. These formulas are not, for the most part, invariable. With patience, you can get them exactly right not only for your general skin type but for your own special skin.

I recommend cold-pressed oils, which, because they have never been heated, retain a higher percentage of natural vitamins; they are available in health food stores and some supermarkets. Also, you should realize that a number of natural oils are completely interchangeable, so you can use the one with the smell that pleases you—or the one you happen to have in the kitchen. Oils in this group are: safflower, sunflower, sesame, and corn oils, as well as cottonseed, linseed, peanut, and almond oils. *Never,* however, interchange olive oil, or the still richer avocado and wheat-germ oils, with any of the others. They are simply too much for all but the driest skins.

Finally, a word about water. Tap water and well water can both contain minerals that you don't want to have in certain preparations; boil it first, or use distilled water. This is especially true in hard water areas, or where water supplies are fluoridated or chlorinated.

STORAGE

One of the reasons why you've decided to make your own products is that you won't have to worry about purity or freshness. As a result, you'll have to pay close attention to the bottles and jars you use to sort and store not only finished products, but raw materials as well. Only glass, porcelain, and stainless steel bottles and jars should be used; finished products, especially, should never be stored in plastic containers, which may contain coloring agents and plasticizers that could contaminate these products. Opaque—or at least dark—glass bottles will also help to protect products (especially nonrefrigerated ones) from deterioration from light. Of course, all nonrefrigerated products should be stored in a cool, dark place.

Gummed labels are a must. Never keep *anything*—raw ingredient or finished product—unlabeled. Include on the label not only the formula's name, but the date it was prepared and any unusual instructions for use. A formula file or notebook is also a good idea, and will prove especially helpful when you find yourself modifying formulas to suit degree of oiliness or dryness, even within a given skin type. It will also help you keep track of seasonal variations, and monitor changes that may be taking place within your skin from year to year.

Be mindful that not all formulations are equally durable. Fresh fruit- and vegetable-based ones are especially perishable, and will keep best when refrigerated, especially since you're refraining from adding any preservatives. If you make a large quantity of a preparation that you use a lot of—body lotion, for instance—employ more than one jar to store it in, e.g., two eight-ounce jars rather than one sixteen-ounce one; that way, you won't risk contaminating the whole batch with bacteria when you dip into it. A fresh jar, capped, unopened, will stand ready—and pure—when you need it; and you should consider using a spatula to spoon out the quantities you'll require for the week's regimen.

All that said, let's turn to the formulas themselves. We'll

go in order of skin type: first dry (and dehydrated); then oily; finally normal (and combination). Formulations appropriate to all skin types will follow. Any "special-interest" formulations, again independent of skin-type needs, conclude the section.

FOR DRY AND DEHYDRATED SKIN
Cleansing Lotions

#1

Cucumber juice	2 cups
Alcohol or vodka	5 tablespoons
Mineral water	1 tablespoon
Honey	2 tablespoons
Egg (whole)	1

Prepare cucumber juice by peeling cucumber, then cutting in slices and liquefying in a blender. Don't worry about the seeds. Strain through cheesecloth, and return to blender. Add all other ingredients and blend until smooth. *Refrigerate.*

#2

Mineral water	1 cup
Alcohol or vodka	2 tablespoons
Witch hazel	2 tablespoons
Glycerine	½-1 teaspoon
Talcum powder	¼ teaspoon

Mix the first four ingredients together. Then add the talcum powder. Shake before using. Need not be refrigerated.

Super-Rich Soaps

#1   Ivory Flakes   1 cup
                   Glycerine   ¼ cup
                Cod liver oil   5 drops

Mix Ivory Flakes and glycerine together with a spatula. Place in a double boiler, and as the mixture begins to melt, add the cod liver oil.

Continue heating until the mixture is thickened, then remove from heat and set aside to cool. When cooled, shape into a circle or an oval with the palms of your hands and leave overnight in a dish or on a piece of foil. This soap will not harden entirely.

#2   Ivory Flakes   2 cups
                 Warm water   1 cup
                   Glycerine   ⅓ cup

Mix together the Ivory Flakes and water with a spatula, then place in top of double boiler and heat until the mixture begins to dissolve. Then add glycerine. Heat until mixture has thickened. Set aside to cool and then roll into a circle or oval shape with the palms of your hands. Leave overnight. This soap has a softer consistency than Super-Rich Soap #1.

Before/After Shave Moisturizers

#1
Mineral water	1 cup
Witch hazel	½ cup
Sesame oil	⅓ cup

Mix all ingredients together and shake before using. Optionally, you can add a few capsules of vitamins A, D, or E, or a teaspoon of liquid lecithin for added emollience and protection.

WATER PHASE:

#2
Borax	2 tablespoons
Water	4½ cups
Witch hazel	¼ cup

Prepare a sodium borate solution by dissolving the 2 tablespoons borax in the 4½ cups water. Bring to a boil and allow to cool. Add 1 cup of the cooled sodium borate solution to the witch hazel. (The remaining sodium borate solution can be stored for future use.)

OIL PHASE:
Beeswax, melted	½ cup
Corn oil	1 cup
Lecithin	1 teaspoon

Melt the three ingredients together in an enameled or glass pot over boiling water.

Mix the oil phase with the water phase in a medium-sized bowl until a smooth, creamy emulsion is obtained. Store in a wide-mouthed 16-ounce jar or, preferably, in two 8-ounce jars.

Protective Cream

WATER PHASE:

Borax	2 tablespoons
Water	4½ cups
Witch hazel	¼ cup

Place borax and water in a pot and boil until the borax is dissolved. Set aside to cool. Then mix 1⅔ cups of the sodium borate solution with the ¼ cup of witch hazel. (The rest of the sodium borate solution can be stored in a jar and kept for future use. It need not be refrigerated.)

OIL PHASE:

Lecithin	⅓ cup
Stearic acid	¼ cup
Corn oil	3 tablespoons

Mix the oil phase ingredients together in a separate pot and heat, over a low flame, until the stearic acid has completely melted. Add the water phase to the hot oil phase and beat with an electric beater until a smooth texture is obtained. Allow to cool, and pour into a 16-ounce bottle or two 8-ounce bottles. Store in a cool, dry place.

Cleansing Cream

WATER PHASE:

Borax   1 teaspoon
Water   1 cup + 1 ounce

Prepare a sodium solution by dissolving the 1 teaspoon borax in the water and bringing to a boil. Allow to cool. (Sodium borate solution may be stored for future use.)

OIL PHASE:

Beeswax, melted   ½ cup
Mineral oil   1 cup + 1 ounce

Melt the two ingredients together in the top of a double boiler.

When they're melted, slowly add 1 teaspoon of the sodium borate solution, mixing with an electric beater until a creamy, smooth mixture is obtained. When it's cooled, store in a wide-mouthed 16-ounce jar or two 8-ounce jars.

Vitamin Night Cream

Stearic acid   1 teaspoon
Lanolin anhydrous   1 tablespoon
Beeswax   2 teaspoons
Peanut oil   1 tablespoon + 2 teaspoons
Water or mineral water   2 teaspoons
Honey   1 tablespoon

Melt all ingredients together over very low heat. When it's cool, add several capsules of Vitamins A, D, and E. Store in a small jar.

After-Shave Masks

#1   Cucumber juice   1 tablespoon
             Kaolin or Dolomite   1 teaspoon
                      Honey   ½ teaspoon

Mix together to form a paste. Apply to face and leave for five to fifteen minutes. Rinse off with lukewarm water.

#2   Mashed strawberries   2
             Talcum powder   1 teaspoon
             Sour cream   1 teaspoon

Mix together with a spoon.

#3   Egg yolk   1
                      Honey   ½ teaspoon
                    Corn oil   1 teaspoon
                   Dolomite   ½ teaspoon

Mix egg and oil by adding oil to the yolk drop by drop. Then add the honey; then the dolomite.

#4   At-home mask   2 tablespoons (*see page* 206)
             Strong chamomile tea   Enough to make a paste

This is a particularly good after-shave mask because of its calming and soothing properties.

FOR DEHYDRATED SKIN
#5   Grated cucumber   2 tablespoons
             Corn or sesame oil   ½ teaspoon
             At-home Powder   Enough to make a paste of medium consistency.

#6   Kaolin or Dolomite   4 teaspoons
            Magnesium carbonate   1 teaspoon
        Cornstarch or arrowroot   1 teaspoon
                         Water   Enough to make a paste

Wheat Bran Superficial Peeling

            Kaolin   2 teaspoons
    Wheat bran (fine)   2 teaspoons
    Water or chamomile
                 tea   2 teaspoons

Mix the three ingredients together to form a medium paste. Apply to skin, *avoiding the eye area,* and leave for five minutes. Then rub all over face using brisk but light circular movements of the fingertips for no more than two or three minutes. Rinse with lukewarm water.

Warm Wax Mask

        Paraffin wax   ⅓ cup
        Mineral oil   ¼ cup
            Lanolin   ⅓ cup
            Beeswax   1 tablespoon
    Crisco shortening   ⅓ cup

Melt ingredients together in a small pot over low heat. When they're melted, test a little of the wax on the inside of your wrist to make sure it is not too hot. Apply throughout the eye area with a brush. Before application, it is necessary to prepare this area by spreading a generous layer of night cream over it. After about 15 minutes, the wax will have hardened, and can be removed by gently easing off with a rubber spatula. This mask is excellent for temporarily eliminating superficial wrinkles and lines.

FOR OILY SKIN

For very oily skin, the following procedure is most helpful. You will need two solutions. First, one cup of water plus ½ teaspoon of borax or sodium bicarbonate. Second, one cup of water plus one teaspoon of lemon juice or vinegar. First clean the face with the borax or bicarbonate solution. After half an hour, rinse off with the lemon juice or vinegar solution.

Cleansing Lotions

#1	Grapefruit juice	½ cup
	Isopropyl alcohol	½ cup
	Witch hazel	¼ cup

Place all ingredients together in a bottle and shake to blend. Instead of grapefruit juice, you may substitute apple juice, which will be more soothing because of its pectin content.

#2	Lemon juice	1 teaspoon
	Vodka	1 cup
	Mineral or tap water	⅓ cup

Place all ingredients together in a bottle and shake to blend.

#3	Egg whites	2
	Lemon juice	3 ounces
	Alcohol or vodka	1 tablespoon
	Tincture of benzoin	1 teaspoon

This will help tighten the pores. Beat egg whites until frothy. In a separate bowl, mix the lemon juice, alcohol, and tincture of benzoin. Pour this mixture slowly over the beaten egg whites and mix well. *Refrigerate.*

#4   Lactic acid   ½ teaspoon
                       Boric acid   ½ teaspoon
                             Alum   ¼ teaspoon
                            Water   1 pint (16 oz.)
       Isopropyl alcohol or vodka   1 cup

Mix the boric acid with the water and boil until the acid is dissolved.
Leave until cool. Then add the lactic acid and the alum. Finally add
the alcohol or vodka.

After-Shave Moisturizers

#1   Yogurt   ½ cup
                        Sea salt   one pinch

Mix and allow the sea salt to dissolve. Can be used as a moisturizer
or a cleanser.

#2   Rosewater   1 cup
                       Glycerine   ¼ teaspoon
             Tincture of benzoin   10 drops

Mix the rosewater and glycerine; then add the tincture of benzoin.

Quince Seed Moisturizer

OIL PHASE:

#3   Stearic acid   ⅔ cup
    Light mineral oil (baby oil)   ¾ cup
                   Paraffin wax   1 tablespoon

Melt all four ingredients over low heat.

WATER PHASE:

          Sodium borate solution   7 cups
             Quince seeds, dried   3 tablespoons

Boil quince seeds in 4 cups of plain water for half an hour, or until a gel-like solution is obtained. While it's still hot, strain through cheesecloth.

Dissolve ⅔ cup sodium borate (borax) with 7 cups plain water by boiling together to make the 7 cups of sodium borate solution. Add this solution to the quince seed gel, and add more water so that the final water phase comes to 9 cups of liquid. Set aside to cool.

Pour the hot oil phase into a larger pot, and slowly add the water phase. Stir with an electric mixer at high speed until all liquid is absorbed and a creamy, smooth emulsion is obtained. Place in jars and refrigerate.

The mild alkalis of this moisturizer are very useful for seborrheic skin and also for mild acne.

After-Shave Masks

FOR LARGE PORES

#1		
	Brewer's yeast	1 teaspoon
	Lemon juice	1 teaspoon
	Honey	1 teaspoon

Blend to a paste, apply, and leave on for five to fifteen minutes. Rinse off with lukewarm water.

#2		
	Kaolin	3 tablespoons
	Cornstarch	1 tablespoon
	Zinc oxide	½ teaspoon
	Magnesium carbonate (optional)	½ teaspoon
	Vinegar	¼ teaspoon
	Water	Enough to mix to paste consistency

Mix the powders; then add the vinegar and water. Apply and leave on for five to fifteen minutes. Very good for soothing inflammations.

#3   Blend mashed avocado with mineral water for an excellent mask to control and moisturize oily skin.

#4

Kaolin	2 tablespoons	
Alum	pinch	
Lemon juice	¼ teaspoon	
Glycerine	½ teaspoon	
Water	Enough to make a paste	

Dissolve the alum in 2 tablespoons of water. Then add the lemon juice and glycerine. Add the kaolin or clay and more water as necessary to make a paste of medium consistency.

#5

Kaolin	2 tablespoons
Glycerine	½ teaspoon
Tincture of benzoin	10 drops
Water	Enough to make a paste

Mix the glycerine and water with the kaolin; then add the tincture of benzoin.

Cornmeal Superficial Peeling

Egg white	1
Cornmeal	2 teaspoons

Mix together and apply on a clean face. When it starts to dry, rub all over face using brisk but light circular movements of the fingertips for no more than two or three minutes, and avoiding the eye areas. Rinse with lukewarm water.

Eye Cream

Use wheat-germ oil, peanut oil, or coconut oil as an eye cream. For added moisturizing, you can add a little liquid lecithin to any of these oils.

Powder for Blackheads

Oatmeal	1 pound
Almond meal or almonds	8 ounces
Orris root	4 ounces
Castile soap	1 ounce

Chip the castile soap into little pieces, and blend with the other ingredients. Place them, little by little if necessary, in a blender, and blend until they are powdered. This mixture can be stored for a year in a cool, dry place. To use, take one or two tablespoonfuls of the mixture and mix with enough hot water to make a medium paste. Rub into blackheads with fingertips, using light, brisk circular movements, then rinse with cold water. Can also be used as a peeling for all skin types instead of the other formulae.

FOR NORMAL AND COMBINATION SKIN

Cleansing Lotions

#1

Witch hazel	1 cup
Spirits of camphor	1 teaspoon
Honey or glycerine	1 teaspoon
Rosewater or orange flower water	¼ cup

Place all ingredients in a bottle and shake well to blend. Need not be refrigerated.

#2

Cucumber juice	1 tablespoon
Lemon juice	½ teaspoon
Boric acid	¼ teaspoon
Vodka	4 ounces
Water	1 pint (16 oz.)

Dissolve the boric acid in the water by boiling together. Let cool, then add the rest of the ingredients.

#3   Honey   ½ teaspoon
                  Rosewater   12 ounces
                      Vodka   2 ounces

Place all ingredients in a bottle and shake well to blend. Need not
be refrigerated.

Before/After Shave Moisturizer

                 Egg yolks   2
                Sesame oil   4 ounces
        Boric acid solution   4 ounces
        Isopropyl alcohol   2 ounces
                 Glycerine   1 ounce

Mix the oil with the egg yolks by adding it drop by drop while stirring with a wire whisk. Prepare boric acid solution as follows: mix
½ teaspoon of boric acid with one pint of water. Boil until the acid
is dissolved. Let cool. Add four ounces (½ cup) to the egg yolk
mixture, and leave the rest for future use. Then add the alcohol (or
vodka) and glycerine. Place in a bottle and mix. Kept in a cool
place, this will last for a month without refrigeration.

Protective Cream

OIL PHASE:

              Liquid lecithin   ⅓ cup
                 Stearic acid   ¼ cup
    Cottonseed or sesame oil   3 tablespoons

WATER PHASE:

        Sodium borate solution   1⅔ cups
                  Witch hazel   ¼ cup

First, prepare sodium borate solution by dissolving 2 tablespoons
borax in 4½ cups of plain water. Boil and let cool. Remainder of solution can be stored in a jar for future use. Heat the oil phase until

all ingredients are liquid and the stearic acid has completely melted. Add the water phase, and beat with an electric mixer until a thin, smooth substance is obtained. Let cool, and pour into jars.

Cleansing Cream (for Combination Skin)

OIL PHASE:

Beeswax, melted	1 tablespoon
Paraffin wax, melted	1 tablespoon
Mineral oil, heavy	¼ cup
Stearic acid	1 tablespoon

Combine ingredients and melt in a medium-sized enamel pot over boiling water.

WATER PHASE:

Sodium borate solution	3 teaspoons

Prepare sodium borate solution by dissolving 3 teaspoons sodium borate (borax) in 1¼ cups plain water and bringing to a boil. Let cool.

Add water phase to oil phase mixing with an electric hand mixer until a smooth liquid-form solution is obtained. Cool and pour into a wide-mouthed bottle.

Night Cream

Cocoa butter	1 tablespoon
Almond oil	3 tablespoons
Lanolin	2 tablespoons
Rose water	2 teaspoons
Honey	½ teaspoon

Melt the first three ingredients over very low heat; then add the rose water and honey. When cool, pour into a jar. To be used only on dry areas, such as the neck and around the eyes.

Wheat Bran Superficial Peeling

Kaolin	2 teaspoons
Wheat bran (fine)	2 teaspoons
Water or Chamomile tea	2 teaspoons

Mix the three ingredients together to form a medium paste. Apply to skin, *avoiding the eye areas,* and leave for five minutes. Then rub all over face using brisk but light circular movements of the fingertips for no more than two or three minutes. Rinse with lukewarm water.

Masks

#1

Rice flour	1 tablespoon
Honey	½ teaspoon
Water	Enough to make a paste

#2

Almonds, finely ground	½ cup
Egg white	1
Rose water or orange flower water	Enough to make a paste

Double Mask (for oily areas such as the "T-zone").
Grind almonds in blender; then mix with egg white and rose or orange water. Can be stored in refrigerator.

#3

Almonds, finely ground	½ cup
Almond oil	3 ounces
Strawberry juice or rose water	Enough to make a paste

(For dry areas of the face).
Grind almonds in blender; then mix with oil and juice or water.

#4   Kaolin   1 tablespoon
        Water, milk, strawberry
        juice, or chamomile tea   Enough to make a paste

If you make this mask with superconcentrated chamomile tea, it
will be very calming for use after shaving.

FOR ALL SKIN TYPES
Eye Cream

            Lanolin   1 tablespoon
        Almond oil   2 tablespoons
       Cocoa Butter   1 tablespoon

Combine ingredients in a small pot and heat over low heat until
melted. Stir, and pour into a small jar.

AT-HOME POWDER MASK FOR VARIOUS SKIN TYPES

        Kaolin or Dolomite
        Calcium carbonate   in equal parts to suit your
       Magnesium carbonate   requirements

When mixed with other ingredients (as follows) and a liquid to
make a paste, the mask is applied to the face and allowed to remain
there for twenty or thirty minutes. It is then removed with tepid
water, leaving the skin soft, firm, and velvety. By stimulating the
circulation of blood, cleansing the pores and then closing them, and
assuring the proper alkaline/acidity level of the skin, this mask
helps the skin to acquire that clear, translucent, glowing look. For
best results, use at least once a week.

    This wonderful mask has many "beautifying" qualities in addi-
tion to the ones stated above—the advantages obtained by being
able to adapt itself for use on numerous types of skin—dry skin, oily
skin, dehydrated skin, sensitive skin, skin with broken capillaries,
and skin with acne problems.

    In each of the following preparations remember to *first* measure one tablespoon of at-home powder into a small bowl, then add slowly little by little the other ingredients recommended for your particular type of skin until there is a paste consistency.

For Dry Skins

1. One egg yolk with small amount of linseed oil (rich in unsaturated fatty acids)
2. One teaspoon of powdered brewer's yeast with one teaspoon of honey and small amount of skimmed milk
3. One tablespoon of powdered brewers' yeast with small amount of linseed oil
4. Appropriate amount of chamomile tea
5. Appropriate amount of sour cream
6. One small slice of a banana mashed with one teaspoon of honey
7. Appropriate amount of skimmed milk
8. Appropriate amount of honey

For Oily Skins

1. One tablespoon of powdered brewers' yeast with small amount of witch hazel
2. Appropriate amount of fresh prune, peach, or apricot juice
3. Appropriate amount of fresh quince juice
4. Appropriate amount of fresh tomato juice
5. Appropriate amount of fresh orange juice
6. Appropriate amount of fresh lemon juice (diluted with water)

For Dehydrated Skins

1. Appropriate amount of fresh canteloupe juice, chamomile tea, or cucumber juice

For Broken Capillaries

1. Appropriate amount of fresh apricot juice (contains Vitamins P and C)
2. Appropriate amount of fresh cabbage juice

3. Appropriate amount of fresh orange juice
4. Appropriate amount of fresh parsley juice or tea
5. Appropriate amount of rosehip tea
6. Appropriate amount of fresh green pepper juice with a few drops of clear honey

For Acne Problems

VITAMIN A APPLICATION:

1. Appropriate amount of fresh carrot juice with small amount of raw spinach extract
2. Appropriate amount of fresh green lettuce juice
3. Appropriate amount of fresh tomato juice
4. Appropriate amount of buttermilk
5. Appropriate amount of mint tea

VITAMIN D APPLICATION:

One teaspoon of powdered brewers' yeast with appropriate amount of above-mentioned fresh juices

VITAMIN C APPLICATION:

Small amount of grated lemon rind combined with the following:
1. Appropriate amount of fresh parsley and/or green pepper juice
2. Appropriate amount of fresh strawberry juice
3. Appropriate amount of fresh lemon juice
4. Appropriate amount of fresh orange juice
5. Appropriate amount of mint tea
6. Small amount of horseradish

SHAVING

Shaving Cream

OIL PHASE:

Stearic acid	¾ cup
Mineral oil	¼ cup
Lanolin	2 tablespoons + 1 teaspoon
Cocoa butter	⅓ cup

WATER PHASE:

Borax	2½ tablespoons
Water	7½ cups (60 oz.)
Chamomile extract	2 ounces

Combine the ingredients of the oil phase in a pot and place over low heat until all ingredients are melted. At the same time, heat the borax and water in a separate pot, and stir to make sure the borax is dissolved. Then pour the hot water phase over the oil phase and stir with a hand electric mixer until a creamy emulsion is obtained. Let cool, add the chamomile extract, and mix again. Store in several jars. Need not be refrigerated, but should be kept in a cool place.

Styptic Lotion

Alum	½ teaspoon
Glycerine	20 drops
Water	2 ounces

To make more concentrated, you may double or triple the amount of alum. Mix all ingredients together. Apply with a Q-tip to razor cuts.

After-Shave Powder

Kaolin (do not substitute another clay)	2 tablespoons
Zinc oxide	¾ teaspoon
Magnesium carbonate	½ teaspoon
Talcum powder	I teaspoon

OPTIONAL:

Rice flour or rice starch	I tablespoon

Mix all ingredients together. If you like, you can add a few drops of your cologne, and mix well.

Apply to the face after shaving to soothe and calm the skin.

After-Shave Lotion

Lactic acid	I tablespoon
Boric acid	I teaspoon
Alum	I teaspoon
Camphor	¼ teaspoon
Rubbing alcohol	2 ounces
Mineral water	6 ounces

To obtain *water phase,* dissolve the boric acid in 6 ounces boiling water; let cool. For *alcohol phase,* dissolve camphor in rubbing alcohol; set aside.

When the water phase is completely cooled, add alum and lactic acid. Then mix the two phases together.

ACNE

Special Cleansing Lotion

#1

Witch hazel	½ cup
Vodka	¼ cup
Spirits of camphor	2 teaspoons
Colloidal sulphur	½ teaspoon
Water	3 tablespoons

Combine all ingredients and shake before using. Never use around the eye areas.

#2

Isopropyl alcohol	4 ounces
Water	2 ounces
Spirits of camphor	½ teaspoon
Citric or lactic acid	one pinch
Colloidal sulphur or	
Salicylic acid	½ teaspoon

Combine all ingredients and shake before using. Never use around the eye areas.

Disinfectant Powders

#1

Rice starch	2 tablespoons
Zinc oxide	½ teaspoon
Talcum powder	2 tablespoons
Magnesium carbonate	½ teaspoon
Alum	¼ teaspoon

The alum should be in the form of a fine powder, such as you will find at any drugstore. Mix well with the other powders, making sure there are no lumps and that all ingredients are evenly distributed.

#2 The same as number 1 except that instead of alum ½ teaspoon of colloidal sulphur is used.

After-Shave Mask

Kaolin or other clay	2 tablespoons
Talcum powder	½ teaspoon
Zinc oxide	½ teaspoon
Cornstarch	½ teaspoon
Magnesium carbonate	1 alum, ½ teaoidal sulphur
½	
teaspoon	

To this powder add enough of any of the following liquids to obtain a paste of medium consistency: chamomile tea, mint tea, ordinary black tea, orange or grapefruit juice, witch hazel, fresh carrot juice.

Disincrustation Compress

Bicarbonate of soda	½ teaspoon
Water	½ cup

Zinc Oxide Ointments

#1

Vaseline	2 tablespoons
Zinc oxide	½ teaspoon
Vitamin A	10 drops or 4 capsules

Melt the vasoline in a small pot. Pour it, drop by drop, over the zinc oxide, stirring well until completely amalgamated. Add vitamin A.

#2   Same as above, plus ½ teaspoon of colloidal sulphur.

FOR THE BODY

Suntan Oils

#1

Wheat germ oil	¼ cup
Peanut oil	¼ cup
Liquid lecithin	1 tablespoon

#2   Avocado oil   ½ cup
                  Peanut oil   ½ cup
                     Olive oil   ¼ cup
                 Mineral oil   ¼ cup

Blend all ingredients. These oils act as only a mild sunscreen. Their primary purpose is to prevent dehydration of the skin during sunbathing. For full protection against ultra-violent rays and sunburning, you must use a 5 percent PABA gel, which you can obtain at any drugstore.

Hand Creams

#1   Lanolin   5 tablespoons
                    Vaseline   5 tablespoons
         Vanillin powder   1 pinch

(For very dry hands.) Melt lanolin and vaseline together over a low heat. When cool, add vanillin powder.

#2   Wheat starch   2 tablespoons
                      Water   1 tablespoon
                  Glycerin   5 ounces

Mix the wheat starch and water together until they form a paste; then add the glycerin.

To apply, wash your hands and just pat dry, leaving them moist. Then massage the hand cream into the skin until dry. After the bath, towel-dry lightly and apply while skin is still a bit damp.

Hand and Body Lotion

WATER PHASE:

Borax	2 tablespoons
Water	4½ cups

Prepare a sodium borate solution by dissolving the borax in the water and boiling until the borax is dissolved. You will need only 6 ounces. The rest may be stored for later use.

OIL PHASE:

Glycerine	¼ cup
Cocoa butter	1 tablespoon
Stearic acid	1 tablespoon

Melt all three ingredients together over low heat.

While still hot, pour ¾ cup (6 ounces) of the sodium borate solution into the oil phase pot and immediately pour the combined mixture into a blender. Blend at medium speed until the mixture is thickened. If it forms lumps, reheat and blend again. Pour into an 8-ounce jar and store in a cool dry place.

Hand and Foot Talcs to Counter Perspiration

#1		
	Talcum powder	5 tablespoons
	Zinc oxide	2 tablespoons
	Boric acid	2½ tablespoons

Combine all ingredients.

#2		
	Tannic acid	2 tablespoons
	Zinc oxide	2 tablespoons

#3		
	Talcum powder	4 tablespoons
	Boric acid	1 tablespoon

This powder reduces unpleasant odors and diminishes activity of the sweat glands.

#4	Talcum powder	3 tablespoons
	Zinc oxide	1 ½ tablespoons
	Boric acid	1 teaspoon
	Salicylic acid	½ teaspoon

| #5 | Spirits of camphor | 4 ounces |
| | Salicylic acid | one pinch |

For rinsing feet after bathing.

Foot Bath

To one quart of warm water, add ½ cup of sea salt or ½ cup of white vinegar.

Bath for the Whole Body

Wrap 2 tablespoons of dried rosemary and 1 tablespoon of sweet basil in a square of cheesecloth. Tie up and drop into a hot bath before bathing. Helps cleansing and relaxation with its fresh fragrance. You may also add a teaspoon or so of avocado oil to your bath to counter dehydration.

Shampoo

Take ½ cup of beer and boil it slowly until it is reduced to only ¼ cup. Add to a simple shampoo formula.

Hair Rinses

#1   FOR OILY HAIR

One teaspoon of lemon juice or vinegar to one cup warm water. Use as a final rinse after shampooing.

#2   FOR DRY HAIR

One cup of chamomile tea (2 tablespoons of chamomile flowers simmered in one cup of water) or 1 teaspoon chamomile liquid extract to one cup of water. Use as a final rinse after shampooing.

For Stimulating New Hair Growth

Tincture of capsicum	2 ounces
Water	2 ounces

Mix the two together, and apply sparingly to affected areas of the scalp every morning and evening. If you cannot get tincture of capsicum, you can pretty easily make your own using the following recipe.

Red cayenne pepper	2 ounces
Vodka	one cup

Mix the two ingredients and leave in a warm place, such as a sunlit window, for two weeks. Shake every day. Then strain the mixture through several thicknesses of cheesecloth. You now have your own tincture of capsicum. It is very strong and stimulating to the scalp, and if it should prove too irritating, should be diluted further, or used less frequently. This is *not* a cure for baldness, but it is a remedy that over many years has been used by top scalp experts to stimulate new hair growth, and has shown its value.

For Tired Eyes

Place a warm wet black or chamomile teabag on each eye for 10 or 15 minutes.

Place cotton pads soaked in water with a pinch of sea salt added over the eyes for 10 or 15 minutes.

INDEX

217